OutRage

Out

Rage!

An Oral History

Ian Lucas

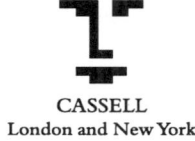

CASSELL
London and New York

> For a catalogue of related titles
> in our Sexual Politics list
> please write to us at an address below

Cassell
Wellington House
125 Strand
London WC2R 0BB

PO Box 605
370 Lexington Avenue
New York, NY 10017–6550

© Ian Lucas 1998

All rights reserved. No part of this publication may be reproduced or transmitted in any form or by any means, electronic or mechanical, including photocopying, recording or any information storage or retrieval system, without prior permission in writing from the publishers.

First published 1998

British Library Cataloguing-in-Publication Data

A catalogue record for this book is available from the British Library

ISBN 0-304-333573 (hardback)
      0-304-333581 (paperback)

Designed and typeset by Ben Cracknell Studios

Printed and bound in Great Britain by
Biddles Ltd, Guildford and King's Lynn

Contents

Acknowledgements vi
Preface: Now Was Not Like That Then ix

1. Pretty Annoyed (But Not Quite OutRaged) 1
2. Coming Out Fighting 13
3. Stolen Kisses, Parting Glances 31
4. Queering the Pitch 49
5. The Whores and the Three-Legged Man 73
6. Sequins, Labia, Children 87
7. Equality Now! 101
8. Another Night of Long Knives 121
9. 'Sister, Sister, It's an Outrage!' 133
10. Music, Cameras, Action! 143
11. Jeans, Genes, Stroppy Queens 159
12. The Riot That Nearly Was 171
13. A Right Holy Row 185
14. Homosexual Terrorists Kill MP 197
15. The Death of Activism? 209

Afterword: Profit and Loss 223

Appendices
1. Chronology 231
2. The Philosophy of OutRage! – An Interview with Peter Tatchell 236

Index 241

Acknowledgements

Boonoonoonoos:
For tea, sympathy, drink, company and memories to all those involved in living and reliving OutRage!:

Adam Jeanes, Ajay, Dice, Alan Jarman, Steve Cook, Fernando Guasch, Keith, Patrick McCann, Lisa Power, Peter Tatchell, Simon Watney, Simon Edge, David Allison, John Beeson, Steve Mayes, Martin Maynard, Dave Arnold, Dave Hurlbert, Marina Cronin, Lynne Sutcliffe, Chris Woods, Steve Stannard, Stuart Colley, Keith Alcorn, Megan Radcliffe, Phil Jones, Edward King, Rob Kemp, Beth Lane, James Kierney, Toby Hopkins, Dave Bunnett, Nick Cave, Graham Knight, John Jackson, as well as Martin and Aamir, Mark Spencer, Edward Pritchard, Sebastian Sandys, Martin Girvin, and Rob Archer who kindly offered time. Credit is also due to Derek Jarman, who offered OutRage! such support, and made me a pot of tea while his apricots soaked.

Many thanks also to those who offered encouragement over the 20-odd months I sat at home in front of my computer and listened to tape after tape after tape. Special thanks to Steve Doherty who bought me a tape recorder and 'broadcast quality' microphone.

For reading and sharing: Cheryl, little brother Paul, Penny Casdagli, Ian Clarke.

Thanks to Alice and Cumbawamba for a picture of Boff in his 'Jason Donovan' T-shirt.

Big thanks to hunky Steve C for looking after this little sister. It wasn't even my idea ...

And for all those homophobes, without whom ...

To
Martin Corbett
and
Simon Kennett
for not going gently into that good night

I don't think my therapist would let me talk about OutRage! ...

ANONYMOUS

A homophobe is a homophobe is a homophobe ... they're all MAAAAAAD!

MARTIN CORBETT

One has only to pick at the scab of memory, and the cries, words and gestures of the past make the whole body of power bleed again.

SITUATIONIST SLOGAN

PREFACE

Now Was Not Like That Then

> It was a dark room. Mirror tiles along the far wall reflected back the faces of sixty-odd, mostly young, queer activists. I was terrified, this being my first attendance at OutRage! They were all so confident, so vibrant, angry and sexy. There was a ripple of anger in the meeting over a queerbashing at a local gay club and all of a sudden we'd decided to go on a spontaneous zap, talking to customers and management. I stood in the OutRage! office donning an OutRage! T-shirt (we only had half a dozen). We were only supposed to borrow the T-shirts for the evening. I never returned mine. The zap was a scream, we knew we were right, the management agreed, it was a nice evening, job well done. I knew I'd be back.

'Now was not like that then' was a phrase I heard on a daytime chat show, used by an irate woman trying to communicate her anger at the loss of values in modern society. Her utter incoherence was hysterically funny, and nobody picked up on the fact that she was talking complete gibberish. Nevertheless, 'now was not like that then' has a ring about it, and I can broadly understand the sentiment behind it.

In the late 1990s, now is not like it was at the beginning of the decade. The canvas is a different colour, a warmer shade of pink perhaps. There are promises of equality before the law, the repeal of Section 28, much gay visibility in the mainstream media, and a burgeoning gay scene. Even the police seem to like us these days.

This book is a series of accounts of what it was like before we got so cosy and popular, and perhaps a glimpse behind the niceties of a more 'tolerant' Britain. Have things really changed so much, or is the new 'tolerance' a thin veneer? Scratch it and see. I write this from Coventry, my home town. Earlier last year, the local gay pub was burned down by arsonists. A gay pub manager was beaten outside his own pub. The local Lord Mayor denounced homosexual 'proclivities', tacitly supported by all his councillors, who failed to show for a launch of a feasibility study into the needs of local lesbian and gay people.

This year, 1998, brings changes good and bad. Lisa Grant loses her case in the European Court against descrimination at work. The 'Bolton Seven' narrowly escape being jailed for consensual gay sex. A Birmingham art student has a book by gay photographer Robert Mapplethorpe confiscated by police for being 'obscene'. For the first time in nearly thirty years, the annual Lesbian and Gay Pride festival is cancelled, after being 'managed' by private enterprise rather than a community initiative. A new national campaign group, Equality Alliance, is formed to coordinate gay activism and lobbying. Peter Tatchell gets arrested for demonstrating against continued religious opposition to gay rights, in Canterbury Cathedral. Labour MP Ann Keen campaigns hard with her out gay son for an equal age of consent. Despite an overwhelming majority in the House of Commons, our quirky democracy allows the House of Lords to oppose it and bully a democratically elected government to drop the amendment from its flasgship Crime and Disorder bill. Meanwhile, over the rainbow, the Government promises to introduce its own bill ensuring an equal age of consent, some 30 years after discrimination was legislated for. Historically, six out gay MPs sit in the Commons. Toto – I've a feeling we're not in Kansas anymore.

This book is the account of Britain's longest surviving lesbian and gay direct action group, told through the eyes of those involved in it. There are 30 or 40 different accounts here, which I have tried to draw together for a coherent account of all their major campaigns and zaps. It's broadly chronological, describing zap by zap, many of which are only directly related in the sense that they involve fighting homophobia, but are not connected with other zaps or actions at the same time. Often, there is friction and disagreement between some of the main protagonists of this story, and I have included different versions while attempting to give as much neutral information as I can. It wasn't all a happy ride by any means.

My own involvement in OutRage! lasted from 1990 until 1994, when I moved out of London. I haven't directly commented on actions I was involved in in the main text of the book – if you want to know what I think, there are some comments in the notes to each chapter. I felt it an advantage to have been involved in the group while researching the book – especially when looking at some of the press reports of what happened, and comparing those to the recollections of the people I interviewed, and my own memories of events. Certainly, when interviewing the many people who agreed to talk about their dark sides for the book, it helped to be an insider.

The personal accounts here are interspersed with some background information, but this has not been an attempt to analyse each and every action, merely to record what went on as truthfully as possible. This seemed particularly important in connection with the more controversial actions such as the FROCS 'hoax' outing, and the outing of Bishops and MPs in 1994/5. This is also very much an account of one group. Other groups, such as Stonewall, Lesbian and Gay Christian Movement, GALOP, Lesbian Avengers, the Sisters of Perpetual Indulgence, are also mentioned here, and have made important contributions in their own right. This account is not a 'fair' history of those groups and is only concerned with them in light of their relationships to OutRage! The focus of the account is also on OutRage! London, but it is important to remember that OutRage! did spawn various local groups, and some of their work is recorded here.

Now was not like that then. It's all change, and nothing's changed. At present, OutRage! is between offices, with a small but committed membership. Earlier last year, Lesbian Avengers stopped meeting and queer activism was declared dead in the gay press. Certainly, it isn't as high profile or as popular as before. Others will debate about its efficacy or importance in the overall picture of gay politics. I have no doubts about its personal and political impact, although others might argue against me. Although I would not stress direct successes from direct action, I think the impact of OutRage! on gay culture, identity, and in raising the profile of lesbian and gay issues is undeniable.

This account ends in 1996. I've included references to campaigns and actions afterwards, but ostensibly the finishing point for this history is the queer political funeral of Martin Corbett in August 1996. I arranged an interview with Martin for this book, but he was unfortunately taken into hospital on the day that we were to meet up. He was one of the founding members of OutRage! and it seems appropriate that an account such as this should close with his funeral, which itself became a political procession and statement. It is a loss for this book that Martin was unable to contribute his account of a project which he spent so much time, energy, vision and strength on. The story of OutRage! that unfolds here was strongly influenced by Martin, and his name appears many times even without him speaking directly. Now was not like that then.

ONE

Pretty Annoyed (But Not Quite OutRaged)

OutRage! was not the first, or only, gay rights activist group in Britain. Other groups had fought for lesbian and gay rights, and employed forms of direct action or activism, albeit for shorter periods of time. Activism in Britain has always been largely a minority sport and gay activism often involved only a handful of people, who would quickly become burned out, and drop out from organizations, which in turn would collapse because of a lack of involvement. Often, lesbian and gay organizations were ripped apart either through internal wrangles (often divided along the lines of race, class or gender) or through external agendas being pursued within the organizations. Both problems would also later beset OutRage!, with serious implications for its organization.

Lesbian and gay activism in Britain had existed for around 20 years before the advent of OutRage! It had existed in different forms and at different times, usually focusing on specific gay-related issues (Section 28 of the Local Government Act, AIDS). Many campaigns had involved personalities who would later go on to join OutRage!, and so OutRage! contained within it the memories of many previous battles lost and won.

Earlier organizations and campaigns had used similar tactics to OutRage!'s media-friendly zaps and campaigns and these were often self-consciously acknowledged by the group. The history of gay activism in Britain is disparate and fractured, with many common threads but no absolute history. Activism itself has been essentially reactive and its history reflects the rise and rise of homophobia, its gains and points of resistance.

Not only did OutRage! need a vision of the future for its actions, but also a sense of the past. The belief in a queer heritage has been used by OutRage! and other queer groups to elicit solidarity and a sense of community and to mobilize support. Along with the rise of queer activism came a renewed interest in queer history and culture, reflected in the increase of publications and media interest in queer sexuality, personalities and events in the early 1990s. The past may be another country, but many members of OutRage! had been natives there at one time or another.

Gay is good – the Gay Liberation Front

The Gay Liberation Front held its first meeting in England in the basement of the London School of Economics on 13 October 1970 and almost immediately became the biggest single influence on homosexual lifestyle of the time. Radically different from the more conservative Campaign for Homosexual Equality, the GLF had been inspired by its American counterpart which had formed as part of the New York counter-culture in 1969.

Having seen the effects of the Gay Liberation movement in the US, the British founders Bob Mellors and Aubrey Walter instigated a movement that followed the American blend of revolutionary politics and alternative lifestyle and which quickly became a significant part of the early 1970s counter-culture. The GLF formulated and published a manifesto in 1971, which was a dialectic blend of radical politics and counter-culture idealism, calling for substantial reorganization of the state and its instruments, most notably gender roles within family and domestic life. The starting point for liberation was 'freeing the head' – throwing off the shackles of self-oppression, and understanding that the personal was political. In 'coming out', as an individual and a gay community, the shackles of oppression could be broken:

We do not intend to ask for anything. We intend to stand firm and assert our basic rights. If this involves violence, it will not be we who initiate this, but those who attempt to stand in our way to freedom.

GLF MANIFESTO[1]

The GLF became known for its loud, controversial protests and lifestyles. The use of street theatre, drag and camp became its trademark and within the short period of its existence the GLF conducted numerous notable and successful protests. Its notorious zap of Mary Whitehouse's Festival of Light in September 1971 – including cross-dressing nuns performing a can-can, the release of white mice, heckling of celebrity speakers Malcolm Muggeridge and Cliff Richard and subsequent challenging of conference attendees – provided both inspiration and a template for future activism.[2] At its height, the GLF involved scores of men and women in political and cultural activity around their sexuality up and down the country, for the first time challenging liberal notions of tolerance with a radical agenda for liberation and sexual revolution.

By 1974, the organization had been largely ripped apart by internal wrangles, political disagreements, and the influence of a changing political scene. Personality clashes, as much as political disagreements, turned a leaderless organization upside down. In splintering, however, the GLF also created many community organizations (Lesbian and Gay Switchboard, *Gay News*, Icebreakers amongst them) which in turn contributed to a strong and visible gay community in London for the first time. An offshoot of the GLF, the GLF Information Service limped on for a number of years distributing information and resources.

The GLF had sparked a feeling of confidence in political sexuality, a public manifestation of what had previously always been locked away in private. It criticized and attacked traditions and establishments which were seen as oppressive, without having to apologize for such attacks. Its legacy would be taken up by many activist groups. When OutRage! was eventually formed in 1990, it was easy and obvious to compare it to its 1970s antecedents. The grass roots organization of the GLF, its spectacular and confrontational zaps and in-your-face celebration of sexuality were important attributes which would be consciously mimicked by OutRage! At the same time, individual members brought with them some of the experiences and knowledge of GLF campaigns and organization. Even before it had disbanded, GLF had rewritten the rules about gay activism and established a political gay constituency which could and would stand against oppression.

[For] some of us, who'd been involved in the Gay Liberation Front like myself, Martin Corbett and John Beeson, [OutRage!] was a bit like reinventing the wheel. There was a sense of *déjà vu*, but a very exciting sense of reinventing something from an earlier, more radical age.

PETER TATCHELL

I had a long argument with Michael Mason, who ran *Capital Gay*. He represented the old GLF – 'you'll never do it, you can never recreate GLF'. There was a lot of cynicism from the old guard, the people who'd seen it before. It had a downside – there was a lot of reinventing the wheel.

CHRIS WOODS

Cosily CHE and going all DAFT

I'd been with the CHE [Campaign for Homosexual Equality] from the age of 19 and that was a bit of an uphill struggle. I suppose I cut my political teeth on it. In CHE, there was an Executive Committee, and you've also got a national membership. People don't feel very involved. The only thing they get is a letter every couple of months or a newsletter.

JOHN JACKSON

Although organizations like the Campaign for Homosexual Equality were campaigning discreetly on lesbian and gay issues, direct action during the late 1970s and early 1980s was *ad hoc* and disparate. The Gay Activists Alliance kept a group of like-minded people loosely in contact with each other in the early 1970s and the formation of gay networks, newsletters and organizations following the split of GLF provided a background of gay community action which would occasionally erupt in a bout of activism, graffiti spray-painting or orchestrated campaigning.

In the early1980s, a group of gay men and lesbian women occasionally met in London as Dykes And Faggots Together (DAFT). Light-hearted and low-key actions were their speciality, more along the line of pranks rather than large-scale public zaps. Typical of such whimsical dares were forays into men-only gay pubs and clubs in order to leave stickers in the loos exclaiming 'A Lesbian Was Here'!

Although it couldn't publicly admit to it at the time, DAFT was also responsible for an infamous prank letter claiming to come from the Department of Employment. Following a comment made by the Archbishop of Canterbury about the possibility of homosexuality being viewed as a disability, DAFT purloined some headed Department of Employment paper, and an unsuspecting DoE employee's telephone extension number. A letter was drafted and sent out to major employers to see what provisions were being made for 'reserve categories of employment' for homosexuals, in line with provisions being made by a new bill for other 'disabled' people.

I thought it was completely obvious what we were about. We were asking whether hairdressing, things like that, should be reserved occupations for homosexuals! People took this horribly seriously – it ended up in the *Mirror* and all sorts. It jammed the Department of Employment's switchboard, all these people phoning up to complain. They thought it was real.

LISA POWER

The DAFT prank, with its sense of mischief and humour, would be mirrored in later OutRage! actions and zaps. Poking fun at institutionalized homophobia and undermining officious busybodies have been some of the light-hearted pastimes of lesbian and gay activists over the past two decades – and a media-friendly way to deflate ill-informed pronouncements by prominent personalities.

Stand up for your love rights – Section 28

By the mid 1980s, 'gay' was being aligned in the popular mind with 'the loony left', the tabloid-created spectre of political correctness gone mad which was intent on spending the hard-earned cash of 'ordinary tax-payers' on fringe groups and minority issues. In October 1987, Prime Minister Margaret Thatcher remarked that 'Children who need to be taught to respect traditional values are being taught that they have an inalienable right to be gay.' On 8 December 1987, MP David Wilshire introduced an amendment to the Local Government Bill, echoing the sentiment of an earlier (failed) Bill of Lord Halsbury aimed at preventing local authorities from 'promoting homosexuality'. The amendment was adopted at the Committee Stage without a vote as Clause 28.

The emergence of Clause 28 coincided with the founding of OLGA (Organization for Lesbian and Gay Action), which arose out of the ashes of a Legislation for Lesbian and Gay Rights Conference at Camden Town Hall. The conference had collapsed in complete acrimony.

My main memory is Peter Tatchell calling up at the end to say something sensible, because everybody else was trying to rip each other's throats out. I ran up to him saying, 'Just put something in the motion to push all this back to the organizing committee to come up with recommendations for further campaigning', just so there was some kind of mandate from the floor – which was terribly important in those days – for somebody to go and do some work. That allowed that committee to start putting OLGA together.

LISA POWER

Feeling immediately under threat as Clause 28 swiftly built momentum within all the political parties, OLGA coordinated a vigorous campaign against the proposed legislation, beginning with a 10,000-strong march in London on 9 January. Thirty-two people were arrested in the course of the protest. Further marches were organized, in London and Manchester. All over the country, walls were spray-painted with anti-Clause 28 graffiti. High-profile zaps, such as a group of lesbians abseiling into the House of Lords, and invading a BBC News studio during a live transmission, highlighted how media 'events' could be used to focus attention on lesbian and gay issues. Contrary to what was being presented in the mainstream media, there were large numbers of politicized lesbians and gay men who were not content to leave politicians to look after their interests.

Clause 28 became Section 28 of the Local Government Act on 24 May 1988. Rather than shutting up the gay community, the effect of the legislation was to give them a voice, and to make it angry. The gloves were now off – the electoral process had absolutely failed lesbians and gay men. More positively, for many people the experience had shown that there was political strength in numbers.³ Section 28 sparked off local and national networks which became the basis for continuing action. Although OLGA itself collapsed (due once more to in-fighting) it had reignited the interest in direct action and activism. Significantly, it brought lesbians and gay men together politically for the first time since the early GLF days. Although it had been forced to respond to the immediate attack of Section 28, OLGA's original intentions had been much more proactive, to campaign for positive legislation on lesbian and gay issues, and on issues of gay identity. Section 28 had altered the perception of gay sexuality – it was an attack on an identified community, not on individuals.

The big success of Section 28 was the direct action, and lesbian involvement in direct action. Those were excellent PR successes, and they reminded everyone how useful that could be. The trouble with Section 28 was that it wasn't backed up by any ability for anybody to go in and negotiate with Parliament. People would not talk to anyone in government. How they thought they were going to alter a government bill, with a sizeable majority, was beyond me!

LISA POWER

My involvement with gay politics began with Clause 28. It was just at the time I was with my first boyfriend, just coming out, and the campaign around Clause 28 I found empowering, liberating and really important in defining myself as an adult gay man.

TOBY HOPKINS

Action equals life – ACT UP London

OLGA was falling apart. It had got itself into a terrible state. There was a spatter of solicitors, accusing people of embezzlement. My girlfriend and I had ceased to go near [the office] because one of the administrators had decided we were agents of the devil. She'd told people she'd seen flames coming out of our heads. It wasn't really a very healthy environment.

LISA POWER

The thing that got me involved in activism, as distinct from writing about it, was ACT UP. One of the things I realized was the interconnectedness between politics and culture that made ACT UP New

York so successful, and the impact that had on people's lives. The other thing I realized in New York, was that I was very angry at the way in which lesbians and gay men were treated in this country.

KEITH ALCORN

The impact of AIDS on the gay community during the 1980s was huge and all-encompassing. Not only did friends and lovers die in great numbers, but the association of a killer plague with queer perverts became fixed in the public mind. Homosexuals were seen as swirling in a cesspit of their own making. That statements such as that could be made by as prominent a figure as Greater Manchester Chief Constable James Anderton were only made more ironic and incredible by the fact that he could claim God told him to say it.

The rise of the 'Moral Majority' in America had led to vilification of people diagnosed with AIDS, and of the wider gay community. In response to continuing government inertia and refusal to deal with what was fast becoming an epidemic, gay writer and activist Larry Kramer founded the AIDS Coalition To Unleash Power (ACT UP) in New York in March 1987. The organization became known for its daring and media-friendly zaps, and it became the focus of many people's expressions of anger. The surge of activism which followed the founding of ACT UP in America articulated a new sensibility within lesbian and gay politics – enough was enough.

Inspired (again) by the American example, in January 1989 more than one hundred people formed a London 'chapter' of ACT UP. ACT UP London quickly became established through a series of high-profile zaps and demonstrations, most notably following the example of its American sister group against major drug companies such as Burroughs Wellcome. The London successes prompted other chapters to start throughout the country, building networks of AIDS activists which – although not campaigning solely on lesbian or gay issues – were largely made up of angry young lesbians and gay men.

ACT UP London shared its offices at the London Lesbian and Gay Centre with OLGA and, later, OutRage! Shared offices meant (sometimes) shared information, but also tension between the groups. Often individuals would be members of both organizations, and divide their time up between them. The groups shared a computer, and having a joint office meant that rent was divided. The demise of OLGA had provided OutRage! with a home and equipment, and a bed-partner in ACT UP.

ACT UP had some very good people, but they weren't the sort who would sit down and organize an office. You tended to get people like Kellan, who'd be sitting at the computer smoking, and putting his cigarette down, and David Allison would come in and say 'You can't smoke around the computer!' We used to have these bloody great notices saying you can't eat around the computer.

JOHN BEESON

ACT UP continued to exist alongside OutRage!, but as OutRage! developed, it stole some of its thunder, and certainly many of its numbers. Many felt that ACT UP London had lost its original direction and became side-tracked into less pressing issues, such as debates about Benetton advertising.[4] A serious financial scandal, resulting in the irrecoverable loss of thousands of pounds, also affected morale, numbers and confidence in the group. For others, OutRage! failed to address the issue of AIDS because they relied on ACT UP to do so; the groups were seen as territorial about their issues. After the closing of the Lesbian and Gay Centre, ACT UP had difficulty finding permanent office space and became increasingly *ad hoc*.

For some of us, the AIDS issues were the most important and most pressing issues for gay activists.

EDWARD KING

[OutRage!] would always argue it wasn't their place, it was ACT UP's, which I thought was ludicrous. It's like saying 'let's privatize the gay community, you deal with that and we'll deal with this bit!' That was one of the reasons, in the end, why I left.

ADAM JEANES

I was very frustrated with ACT UP, because I felt it was still stuck in a political model that was very much of the 1970s and '80s, which was very much concerned with equal opportunities politics, being morally right rather than having any sort of political impact.

KEITH ALCORN

ACT UP was becoming a mouthpiece. OutRage! learned something from the dissent that had made ACT UP into much less than it could have been.

SIMON WATNEY

Many of us had been involved in London ACT UP, and saw how direct action could be effective in putting AIDS on the public agenda. We felt it was time to use similar tactics to raise the profile and visibility of lesbian and gay issues.

PETER TATCHELL

Becoming professional homosexuals

It was very clear that Section 28 had been allowed to happen because there was no effective voice against homophobia at the time. There was no respected organization to argue reasonably for legislative reform and articulate arguments in favour of lesbian and gay equality. During the campaign against the clause, a group of activists began to form who felt that they could carry forward some of the work, and build much more effectively for a professional lesbian and gay lobbying group. In addition, the formation of the American lobbying and campaign group the National Gay and Lesbian Task Force in the late 1980s provided a new model for effective and professional homosexual rights campaigning.

I came away from that campaign thinking both of those sides of things had to be revived. [Stonewall] was set up with a defensive structure, to stop it from being taken over by the straight left, which was what kept happening.

LISA POWER

Not everyone saw the group as being self-protective, however. Although Stonewall's broad aims were welcomed, there was suspicion from other sectors of the gay community who believed that the group was giving itself airs and graces, and that it was being run by political hacks and media-hungry minor celebrities. There was also resentment that Stonewall was completely unaccountable, yet could claim to speak for lesbians and gay men.

Spearheaded by actors Ian McKellen and Michael Cashman, Stonewall lay down its brief during the early months of 1989. It would concentrate on drafting a lesbian and gay rights bill, which would also focus attention on the debate around an equal age of consent. The current age then for consensual sex between men was 21, and more than anything it seemed to symbolize the way in which institutionalized homophobia operated.

The establishment of a professional campaigning organization was itself symbolic; it proved that it was possible to challenge homophobia, and to organize solely around lesbian and gay rights. It established the fact that there was popular support, not only within the gay community, but outside of it, for a more assertive stance on equality, and that homosexuality was no longer invisible. For a number of high-profile and powerful personalities, it wasn't just an embarrassment, but a source of pride. A sister charity, the Iris Trust, was also set up to provide funds for education and research. Homosexuality was at last becoming 'respectable'.

Stonewall wasn't a gay organization as we know it. It was much more a small company, talking to Parliamentarians, which nobody had done before. It had been greeted with a huge amount of resentment by the existing right-on professional activists, who were horrified by the 'straightening' of gay activism which it represented. And it did represent that – taking on the straight world, on its own terms.

LISA POWER

By the end of the 1980s, lesbians and gay men in Britain had seen gay rights put firmly back on the political agenda. This was due in large part to the effects of AIDS, which focused much public discussion on sexuality and blame, and which became synonymous with gay identity. Gay became 'Got AIDS Yet?' In addition, the broader political climate was becoming much more conservative, indeed reactionary, in Britain and the United States. President Ronald Reagan and Prime Minister Margaret Thatcher both had strong personal commitments to 'family values'. Firm 'moral' guidance was twinned with strong anti-socialist sentiment, anti-union legislation and a reappraisal of the Welfare State. 'Gay rights' became the bogeyman that united all these threads – it was seen to undermine the family, to bring disease and depravity into society, and to be symptomatic of the worst excesses of far left ideology. Ironically, gay rights were very low on the agenda of far left or revolutionary organizations, who argued that all minor struggles were united in the class struggle, and that gays had to wait for the revolution before liberation.

The 1980s increasingly saw the role of marketing and publicity, and the rapid growth of the media industry. Even the Prime Minister's image was recreated to have a softer tone, a gentler voice to help the harder line. It wasn't just what was said that was important, but how it was said and who said it. The media were looking for stories and personalities which were exciting, contentious and self-contained. It was for this reason that Stonewall had formed, realizing that behind empty political rhetoric lay vast armies of professional image makers, lobbyists, strategists and networkers.

The 1980s had been full of frustration, anger, loss – of people and liberties. Activism and campaigning by lesbians and gay men for lesbian and gay issues were becoming a necessity and new strategies were having to be adopted. The legacy of lesbian and gay campaigns since 1970 had not led to any significant improvement for lesbians or gay men within society. In fact, people were beginning to realise that things had actually became a lot worse.

I had a lot of frustration and anger. If OutRage! hadn't come along, I would have probably gone into bombs or something – damn OutRage! It seemed like a constructive way to direct my fury at culture in general, get back at it!

DAVID ARNOLD

Back home in San Francisco, I'd been involved in grass roots organizing, working mostly with indigent mothers living in derelict public housing. In London I expected that to continue – I wanted to get involved where I might do the most good for the most oppressed. I quickly discovered that the most oppressed group around was my own kind! A giant dose of reality for a gay man from San Francisco!

DAVE HURLBERT

[There was] real distress amongst lesbians and gay men, who'd grown up through the eighties really frightened, deeply, deeply frightened of policing, brutalization, and the life of London in the eighties, which was rough, and violent, and hideous.

SIMON WATNEY

NOTES

1. Extract from the GLF Manifesto, 1971, reprinted in Lisa Power, *No Bath but Plenty of Bubbles: An Oral History of the Gay Liberation Front 1970–73* (Cassell, 1995), p. 330.
2. See Power, *No Bath but Plenty of Bubbles*, for a detailed account of the Festival of Light zap, and account of the rise and fall of GLF.
3. The Clause 28 Campaign was also my own political and personal coming out. I travelled down from Aberystwyth with the local university gaysoc to take part in an Association of London Authorities debate on the clause, where we were applauded as soon as we announced that we were from Wales (bravo to these brave people from the sticks!). In small groups we were encouraged to provide feedback in Welsh, even though only one of us could speak the language. But it added street cred to our arrival there, and everyone else wanted to be seen as good little liberals. I took part in the usual things – debates, spray-painting, marches. On a coach trip back from one of the London marches, we were stopped by the police. Having only managed to half-fill our coach with people, they asked if we could take back passengers from another coach that had broken down. It was a party of men from the local factory's male voice choir. They got on to the coach as 'Male Stripper' by Man2Man was playing, a perfect entrance. It wasn't long before they realized the coach was full of screaming queens, and the lads broke into two camps – the 'backs-against-the-wall gang' who fell asleep on the back seat (despite their best efforts to keep at least one eye open), and the others who would at least talk to us. The general opinion was that no one in their factory could be gay. 'They just couldn't be.' Before leaving, one guy tapped me on the shoulder. 'My brother-in-law's gay, it's all right, we get on great Good luck with the campaign, I hope you make it.' I also wished him well as he and his mates slipped off into the night. 'I met a male stripper in a go-go bar…'
4. I was at a meeting of ACT UP when the Benetton PR team came to 'discuss' the use of a picture featuring David Kirby, a man dying from an AIDS-related illness. They'd dressed in 'rad drag' – leather jackets (obviously just off the peg) and designer jeans. Hoping to look as if they fitted in, their clothes branded them as pseuds. I can remember them saying that they weren't advertising, merely raising issues. I asked if that was the case, why they couldn't put helpline numbers on the posters or ads. Well, that would have been a little too obvious, I guess.

TWO

Coming Out Fighting

OutRage! was conceived as a coalition within lesbian and gay British politics and to insist on a certain level of fun politics in the wake of that tidal wave of homophobia in the eighties. It was about a moment in time.

SIMON WATNEY

Seven years ago, London had a very limited commercial gay scene. Political activity was really restrained, there were two gay newspapers, no gay radio programmes, virtually no discussion of gay issues in the press. There were very few high-profile out lesbians or gay men, there was no discernible area like Old Compton Street.

KEITH ALCORN

It was only a matter of time before there was an eruption of outrage in early 1990. On both sides of the Atlantic, the sport of 'queerbashing' was on the increase, with gay men and lesbians on the receiving end of verbal, political and physical attacks almost daily. A number of vicious attacks on gay men in and out of London became a sinister background to the new year. William Dalziel had been found on the street in West London bleeding from head wounds in January 1990, and later died. Ian Erskine's naked body had been found in a plastic bag in Ely, Cambridgeshire, after he had disappeared from London in December 1989. They were the latest victims in a catalogue of gay-related attacks, which police seemed unable to solve.

At the same time, a number of high-profile police entrapment campaigns, including one at Hyde Park Corner toilets, were seen as an unjustifiable diversion of police resources which, people were beginning to argue, might be better spent in dealing with gay men as victims of crime rather than perpetrators.

At 1.00 a.m. on Monday, 30 April 1990, a 49-year-old actor named Michael Boothe was viciously kicked to death in public toilets in Hanwell, West London, by what he told ambulance staff was a gang of six or seven men. It was one of 14 unresolved gay-related murders dating back to 1986, five of which had happened at 'cruising grounds'. What the police called 'a merciless killing' had almost no witnesses, and although several people were involved, no information could be found relating to the crime.

It immediately focused all the things that we were concerned about into a set of issues that were easy to articulate and which marked a completely new departure in terms of street activism.

KEITH ALCORN

For me, the final straw was reading about the actor who was kicked to death in a public toilet. I determined to do something even if it had to be a single-handed effort.

DAVE HURLBERT

The continued police entrapment campaigns brought their own catalogue of statistics. In 1989, an estimated 5000 gay men had been arrested for consensual same-sex behaviour – the highest amount recorded since the 1950s, before homosexuality had been partially decriminalized.[1]

There was a conjunction of events at the very beginning of May which made it very clear that something like OutRage! was needed. Perhaps if it had happened earlier, it might not have had the same degree of success.

KEITH ALCORN

Queer in America

Following divisions within ACT UP New York, American activists began to develop a new lesbian and gay group, which first met at New York's Community Services Center in March 1990. Queer Nation built activism based on sexual identity – not just lesbian, gay or bisexual, but *queer*. Queer was used as an in-your-face catch-all designer label. Its shocking tone caught some of the violence shown against lesbian and gay communities in America, and threw it right back. It was also a call to queer nationalism – a community that confronted homophobia and had collective responsibility for dismantling the power of 'the closet'.

We felt we'd finally had enough. Something had to be done. We weren't going to be kicked around anymore. We wanted to do something to fight for our lives.

PETER TATCHELL

At the beginning of April, the weekend of the Poll Tax Riot, Michelangelo Signorile[2] came to stay with me. We were talking about the difference between gay politics in New York and gay politics in Britain and it suddenly clicked that the thing that was needed in London was something like Queer Nation. He described the way in which Queer Nation worked and immediately it was clear to me that this was something we could do in London, and that it would work.

KEITH ALCORN

Three queers and a greasy spoon

Queer Nation, and the state of events in Britain, led to three gay men becoming more and more interested in setting up a group to campaign on queer issues in London. Informal chats now became more formalized. Simon Watney, Keith Alcorn and Chris Woods began to look at how their idea might be put into practice.

I was writing for *Capital Gay* and that was how I came to know Chris Woods. We discovered we had a lot of ideas in common, as I did with Simon Watney who was in New York at the time I was there. The thing that we diagnosed as particularly problematic was the unwillingness of many lesbians and gay men to take a political stand.

KEITH ALCORN

So we decided to call a meeting and we sat in this cafe in Gray's Inn Road and mapped out the kind of organization we thought we'd like.

CHRIS WOODS

We decided to call a meeting at the Lesbian and Gay Centre, all the great and the good, the clowns and the jugglers.

SIMON WATNEY

Half the list was people who had been involved in gay politics for some time and half the list was people who hadn't been, but we knew would be really receptive to something like this. Chris and I wrote this letter and then circulated it, had no idea whether anybody would turn up. People began to get really excited by it, calling us up and saying 'oh, can I bring so-and so…?' At this point, we still weren't sure that we wanted to start some sort of organization, but we just wanted to see if there was enough energy around the idea to call a public meeting.

KEITH ALCORN

The meeting for those interested was to be held at the third floor room at the Lesbian and Gay Centre at Cowcross Street in Farringdon, on 10 May. Although not a public meeting, the number of people interested in attending grew and grew until between 40 and 60 people were expected. Without a name or constitution, the group and meeting became known in the gay press as 'The 10th of May' group – until something better came along.

As well as the three 'founding fathers' attending the first meeting, representatives came from the Campaign for Homosexual Equality, GALOP, the gay press, and people who had been involved in pre-Wolfenden lobbying (when homosexuality was completely illegal) and the Gay Liberation Front. Individuals included Gillian Rodgerson, Peter Tatchell, Jean Frazer, Lisa Power, Michael Mason and Martin Corbett. After talking through their reasons for the meeting, Chris, Simon and Keith let events take their own course.

[We] just basically put the idea to them, said 'This is what we're thinking of doing. Do people think it's going to work? What do people think the problems are going to be?'

CHRIS WOODS

We were all united in wanting a group that would specifically focus on direct action for lesbian and gay emancipation. We didn't want to become an all-purpose group fighting on a broad leftist agenda, covering every issue under the sun. There were already plenty of groups doing that. We didn't want to become a political party. We set out to have a very specific and narrowly focused agenda of fighting homophobia.

PETER TATCHELL

At the end, somebody said 'We've got to pay for the room, let's take a collection.' I signed a cheque for the room. I didn't tell anyone. I thought they wouldn't like it because they were very anti-Stonewall. Stonewall paid for that first meeting! I always kept that quiet, and thought it rather funny.

LISA POWER

Getting a name for themselves

After proving that there was indeed a groundswell of opinion in favour of setting up a group, a second meeting was advertised in the gay press, which was open to all members of the public. Held again at the London Lesbian and Gay Centre, the meeting fed off the new energies and anger which arrived with the new recruits.

Very, very quickly, three key people presented themselves, and they were Dave Hurlbert, Shane Broomhall and Steve Stannard, and they immediately took a very important role in driving the group forward.

KEITH ALCORN

I saw the ad in a gay paper. I was inspired. I realized that at last something was going to happen. I remember Peter Tatchell saying early on 'It's not about the class thing it's about gay rights.' Not being in England long, this was incomprehensible – but that statement came back to haunt me throughout my involvement with the group.

DAVE HURLBERT

People were asked to jot down ideas and at the end we would come back and look at the various suggestions. I jotted a brief series of points on the back of an envelope, which was subsequently adopted as the OutRage! aims and objectives. There was quite a big debate in the group about my insertion of the word 'non-violent'. Myself and the majority deliberately inserted the words as a conscious attempt to try and orientate OutRage! away from the macho style of traditional leftist politics and take on board the lessons of the feminist movement. It is necessary to reject violence, which has been a key element in our oppression.

PETER TATCHELL

The group adopted a series of aims and objectives which specifically focused on fighting homophobia, and which put gay rights in the context of civil rights and demanded an agenda which encompassed but went beyond law reform, challenging how society itself viewed and treated homosexuality. The adopted Statement of Aims was:

OutRage! is a broad based group of lesbians and gay men committed to radical non-violent direct action and civil disobedience to:

> Assert the dignity, pride and human rights of lesbians and gay men

Fight homophobia, discrimination and violence against lesbians and gay men

Affirm the right of lesbians and gay men to sexual freedom, choice and self-determination.[3]

The aims and objectives were quickly adopted by the group, and the aims would be read out, almost as a mantra, before every meeting, along with a call for journalists, police officers and representatives of other groups to declare themselves.

Having now established what they were, the '10th of May Group' also needed to be able to say who they were, and so they began to search for a name and an identity.

There were many different suggestions for the name. I can only remember my own unsatisfactory effort which was GAYLE-FORCE – Gay And Lesbian Equality Force!

PETER TATCHELL

In the first week, we had a meeting at our flat, when we came up with the name of 'OutRage!' which was in fact my idea. I used to write for *Outrage* in Melbourne.

SIMON WATNEY

It was me that came up with the name. I can't think what made me think of it, but as soon as I thought of it, I immediately thought 'Yes! That's the name!' It's got to be something that immediately communicates – it did immediately communicate what the group was about.

KEITH ALCORN

The name was meant to symbolize that we were out as lesbians and gays and were filled with rage at the injustices which were perpetrated against us. Together, the word symbolized the outrage we felt about homophobia, and the outrage we intended to cause in fighting back against it.

PETER TATCHELL

My friend Paul drew the logo on the back of a cigarette packet at Simon's [Watney] kitchen table. It also looked like the T-shirt that season that Jean Paul Gaultier was doing, which said 'Gaultier', on the same sort of pattern. It was deliberately referential.

KEITH ALCORN

A clothes shop in Christopher Street is where the logo came from. We went to a meeting and it was approved.

SIMON WATNEY

A piece of the action

By 24 May, OutRage! had a name, a swanky logo, a set of objectives, and a growing membership. As yet, it hadn't done anything. A choice of actions was available. The first action to be seriously discussed was in the light of Ann Winterton's amendment to the draft Human Embryology and Fertilization Bill, which was looking at how fertilization and storage of fertilized embryos should be controlled. Winterton's amendment would have prevented lesbians from gaining access to fertilization treatments. By the time the issue was discussed by OutRage!, the amendment had already failed, and there was no representative to give a report back to the group on the Bill.

The second issue to be discussed was that of policing the gay community. This had been given immediacy by the highly publicized murder of Michael Boothe, a further attack on an 18-year-old student at a cruising ground in Chatham on 5 May, and the murder of a Glaswegian man on 11 May. That an action against the police should take place was not at issue. The type of action was hotly debated, with a number of alternatives put forward. Suggestions for where the action should take place included St James's tube station, New Scotland Yard, in front of the toilets in Hyde Park, and at the Ealing Police headquarters. After a large group discussion, two proposals were forwarded: an action outside New Scotland Yard, or an action at Hyde Park toilets.

The plan was to hold a dignified demonstration with signs, perhaps at Scotland Yard or Parliament. I proposed a different idea: 'We're not going to get any media if we do that, we've got to do something unusual ('outrage-ous') in order to get any coverage. Why don't we demonstrate where the murder occurred? Right there at the toilet!'

DAVE HURLBERT

There was a very clear fissure between people whose model of political activity up until that point had been to go to the institution responsible – no matter how unphotogenic – and on the other side, the people who said 'Yes, let's go to the cottage because it will make fabulous photographs!' Nobody would accuse Peter Tatchell of being camera shy these days, but Peter was one of those who said 'No, we should do it at New Scotland Yard.' It's interesting to see what OutRage! did to him.

KEITH ALCORN

The decision to demonstrate at Hyde Park cottage was carried by 14 votes to 11, with one abstention. The action was planned for Thursday, 7 June, at 1.00 p.m. It had already been intimated that at least one television company, LWT, was interested in the action, and that further media coverage could be encouraged. The Gay London Policing Group (GALOP) were approached to take care of legal coverage, and a decision was made not to inform the police, as the demonstration would not be illegal. It was planned to have a number of placards with pictures of murdered gay men on, with a slogan on each.

On the day, around 35 OutRage! members attended the demonstration, meeting at 12.45 a.m. at Hyde Park tube station. A crew from LWT had indeed shown up, and there was interest from the gay press. The demonstrators posed for photographs in and out of the cottage, and the police profile was generally low. The action was a success, although a later meeting pointed out that afternoon zaps prevented large attendance, more time and care needed to be put into planning events and placards, and that a chief coordinator should be appointed.

There must have been 20 or 30 people outside with placards, walking around, doing mock cruising, generally making a noise. The group felt tremendously empowered, people were really pleased to be out there on the streets doing an action.

TOBY HOPKINS

It was symbolic and terribly important that OutRage! began with a controversial public action around policing and sexuality, and public space and private space. That's the sort of stuff most of us were involved in, not just an airy-fairy postmodernist theory, but concrete issues about legality and sexuality. We managed to get a clear message into the press about policing and crimes without victims, going back to those common-sense issues in a very clear way.

SIMON WATNEY

Right from the beginning, it set a style, and it never really changed from that.

CHRIS WOODS

Even then, perhaps particularly then, people had a sense of history in OutRage! One of the themes of Hyde Park was that we were consciously emulating the first GLF demo, where they went to Highbury to do a cottaging action.

TOBY HOPKINS

Getting it together

At the time of the Hyde Park cottage demonstration, OutRage! had £16 to its name. It was borrowing space from the OLGA /ACT UP shared office at the London Lesbian and Gay Centre, and it didn't have a formal structure. OLGA eventually offered its office space and computer (known affectionately as 'Fluffikins') to OutRage!, and the LLGC Director, Oscar Watson, in an attempt to appease OutRage!'s anxieties about the responsibility of a weekly office rent of £62.50, pointed out that as it would take the Centre a good deal of time to find any new tenants, they would not be thrown out too soon if they could not pay the rent.

An 'office group' began to form, with Martin Corbett following on from his OLGA and GLF roles, joined by John Beeson, David Allison and Adam Jeanes, amongst others. Very quickly, an 'acquisition list' – or a 'Nick List' – was drawn up, made up of the various things that Outrage! needed to beg, borrow or steal, in order to work – stationery, office equipment, furniture. The Office Group began to meet regularly on Sundays, to sort through the administration of the group. The minutes of all meetings were typed and filed, and the new office was staffed on a regular basis.

At the same meeting I joined, David Allison joined. It was all a bit intimidating to walk into – whenever they tried to organize a meeting, they all took out their Filofaxes. They said these are the sub-groups we're setting up. I thought, well, I know nothing about fund-raising, I know nothing about actions, but I do know about offices, so I joined the office group there and then!

ADAM JEANES

I turned up at the office with a sizeable involuntary corporate donation of office essentials, e.g. paper clips staplers, pens, paper, etc. Initially, Martin Corbett and I assumed responsibility for the day-to-day running. I took responsibility for replying to letters, Martin made sure that the office was kept tidy, that papers were filed correctly, and every Sunday afternoon we did the dusting and vacuuming.

DAVID ALLISON

We were constantly looking round skips. I remember looking out a window at the Centre and seeing chairs in a skip on the corner. We all dashed downstairs and got them. They were nice chairs, you could lean back on them, but nobody realized how far you could lean back on them until you fell out!

ADAM JEANES

Our second computer was donated by Michael Mason, of the late and much lamented *Capital Gay*. A gem of a human being, he donated the money anonymously.

DAVID ALLISON

Money, money, money

Once OutRage! started to do things, it became very apparent that actions would cost. Materials were needed to make placards, send out press releases, create costumes and props, as well as to keep the office working and the Thursday meetings going. A fundraising group was set up to raise money for the group. Following a suggestion by Dave Hurlbert, a collection was taken up during Thursday meetings and managed to raise some funds to keep the group afloat. However, it was clear that more imaginative ideas would be needed.

OutRage! set up a bank account, based in a bank branch where one of its co-treasurers, Steve Stannard, worked. Two treasurers, Steve and a courier called Mike Burgess, were elected as co-treasurers, with OutRage! now functioning as a not-for-profit organization. It was also beginning to use its media-friendly image and know-how to create imaginative ways of raising money, through the sale of OutRage! merchandise.

I brought back a design from a New York artist called Adam Rawlston, of the 'I Am Out Therefore I Am' T-shirt, which I had seen in New York. He said 'Yes, you can have it as a fundraising thing.' I had some money so I put up the money to print however many for Pride, and we sold virtually all of them.

KEITH ALCORN

I wanted to lay a pink triangle on the Cenotaph on the morning of Pride. I made thousands of pink poppies, and the idea was to give them away to people or ask for donations, to pay for the wreath. It was obvious, because lots of people got involved, that it was going to make far more money than was needed. I was looking for something to give the money to, went along to a meeting, explained what I was doing, asked if

OutRage! wanted the money, and they said 'Yes!' and were quite positive about it.

DAVE BUNNETT

There were suggestions that OutRage! should set up sex lines, and that we would then get the rake-off. It was a serious suggestion, that you would have these sex lines, saying 'this is promoted by OutRage!, an organization that fights against discrimination against lesbians and gay men,' and then someone would listen to whatever wank message they wanted to, and spend their 49 pence. For many of us it was outrageous, an unprincipled way of making money.

STEVE STANNARD

I did a lot of fundraising. The first meeting I went along to, I went with my friend Alan, and Alan's big ambition in going along to OutRage! was to discover what Simon Watney's wallpaper was like. Simon said he was going to have a fundraising meeting at his house, and so Alan and I said we'd go along to the Fundraising Group! Simon was a very good host, and we rather liked his decor!

TOBY HOPKINS

The selling of OutRage! T-shirts (at £6 each, £8 through retail stores such as Gay's the Word) was immensely successful. They sold on the fact that it was cool to be queer, and acted as publicity for the group, as well as badges of affiliation and identity for the wearer. OutRage! was not only being mentioned in the papers, but its visibility was enhanced by its logo appearing on people's chests in the streets. OutRage! was fashionable, and fashion-conscious.

With anti-gay violence in the background, OutRage! hit upon a scheme which allowed queers to believe that they were doing something to stop the violence, to foster a sense of community, to give another queer ID badge to wear, and to have some fun. On a trial basis, £50 was set aside to buy 150 whistles.

In New York they were encouraging people to carry whistles. The idea behind the whistle was not just something you could use to call for help, it was also a sign, in the same way as a red ribbon. I hit upon the idea that we could sell the whistles as a fundraising thing. We made a fucking fortune in the first few months that we were doing it. The other huge benefit was that it allowed us to go out and talk to people about what we were doing and why we were doing it. The whistle patrols were one of the most important early actions that OutRage! did. They were important in terms of outreaching to other people, they were important in terms of bonding groups together – people did them as a social thing.

They were important in giving people with very developed ideas about where OutRage! was going a chance to put those across to people who'd just come into the group, and effectively to indoctrinate them. It also gave people a chance to get off with each other.

KEITH ALCORN

I got the first whistles. I went out and got a dozen whistles – I think the first dozen were to blow on demonstrations. They were very popular and at the same time the club scene was moving from high energy to techno, and the whistles were really big for blowing on the dance floor. You'd go into a club and it would be peaceful, and by the time you'd left, there'd just be a pandemonium of noise.

TOBY HOPKINS

We were more successful in raising money than any other lesbian or gay people I've ever met, in such a short space of time. Those organizing whistle patrols were making it very clear it wasn't about selling whistles at all. Actually, it was about raising people's awareness of OutRage! being around. OutRage! raised the profile of violence against lesbians and gay men more than anything else that's happened, really. Everyone we know has been affected by violence in one way or another.

STEVE STANNARD

There was a little leaflet attached to the string. People met earlier on a Friday night at the Centre and then went off selling whistles.

AJAY

People wanted to give OutRage! money, because they'd done some noisy actions and they saw it was something that wanted to protect their community, and there was a huge amount of good will towards them.

LISA POWER

I remember going on a whistle patrol to Brighton. It was so funny because we went to Club Revenge, and they'd got a security thing where if there was any trouble they'd blow whistles at each other. So they didn't know we were in the club selling whistles. With 300 queens, what are they going to do? They're going to blow their whistles! So the music kept getting turned off and the lights kept going up. Obviously the managers clicked on to this, and said 'If anyone blows their whistles, they're going to be kicked out.' Obviously you say that to queens and they all blow their whistles!

JAMES KIERNEY

The whistles were cheap to buy, Day-Glo coloured plastic attached to brightly coloured shoe laces, tied in a safety knot which could be ripped off to prevent choking. They became a feature of nearly all OutRage! demonstrations, and standard fare on Pride marches. The fundraising group also realized the vulnerability of volunteers with collecting tins and instigated a system of sealing and signing for the tins. By mid 1990, only a few months after its inception, OutRage! had a very sound financial footing.

Trashing and cashing in at Pride

With Pride looming, the OutRage! PR and fundraising machine went into overdrive. At Pride itself on 30 June, OutRage! had its own stall with leaflets and merchandise, staffed by volunteers and OutRage! members keen to publicize the group. The 7'× 3' stall cost £35. On the day of Pride, OutRage! became involved in a more controversial action, when individual members identified a target within the Pride Festival itself.

At the time, a booklet produced in 1987 by two members of the Revolutionary Communist Party, Dr Michael Fitzpatrick and Don Milligan, titled *The Truth about the AIDS Panic*, was questioning the way in which safer-sex messages were being delivered by the gay community, in the light of a government-created 'panic' about AIDS. The pamphlet claimed that AIDS activists were colluding in the oppression of homosexuals by preaching 'safer sex' without challenging the wider discrimination against homosexuals, and also questioned the reality of HIV being responsible for AIDS.

The RCP had their own stall at Pride, which was attacked and picketed by several OutRage! members, but was not officially a planned OutRage! action. The spontaneous zap became a focus point in uncovering political and personality differences within the group, and underlying tensions became significantly more tangible when the action became known.

The RCP's line was there was no epidemic whatsoever, in any shape or form. It was a particular brand of leftism that objected to self-organization of any type. A group of us, in a fairly *ad hoc* way on the day, thought we ought not to sit back. People wandered over to the RCP stall. Maureen Oliver had the megaphone at one point, and stood at the stall and denounced them. They didn't know what to do, they didn't respond much. Then the group dispersed.

EDWARD KING

[The RCP] were merely questioning the HIV Equals AIDS idea. Simon Watney had intended long before the day that he would do that. There were two OutRage! activists who refused to take part in it. It was quite unacceptable for him to regard that as a spontaneous zap by OutRage! We hadn't discussed what our attitude on HIV/AIDS was. It was the use of the OutRage! name by Simon Watney because he'd been involved in setting it up.

STEVE STANNARD

They did fuck up the stall, they did overturn it. [Simon] was very distraught because he was getting a lot of flack and he said to me 'David, we've been friends for twenty years, you don't think I'm a fascist, do you?' I said, 'What do you mean, friends? You've barely said hello to me in the last twelve years!' and walked off. It hadn't been raised at a meeting. If it had, I'd have argued vigorously against doing anything at all. I think probably the RCP are much closer to the truth than GMFA [Gay Men Fighting AIDS].

DAVE BUNNETT

March for Michael Boothe

The most immediate and tangible expression of anti-gay violence had been the murder of Michael Boothe in Ealing. It wasn't only OutRage! that had taken an interest in the murder; local gay men had come together under the Ealing Lesbian and Gay Forum in order to hold a public observance of Michael Boothe's murder at Elthorne Park, followed by a march to the Town Hall. A representative from the group had approached OutRage! on 31 May 1990 to enlist support.

On 10 July, a couple of hundred people joined the march. There was a brief fracas when a spectator attempted to cause a disturbance, but otherwise the march was dignified, though angry. Shane Broomhall and Peter Tatchell both made speeches at the Town Hall, and OutRage!'s own leaflets were distributed and T-shirts sold.

It was the first action at which OutRage! was visible, and we had a banner. My recollection, more than anything else, was the degree of tension at our presence there.

KEITH ALCORN

We weren't leading things, but we were running into wider networks of concerns and wider networks of anger. I remember the people organizing the Michael Boothe group were feeding into the demonstrations that were happening at that time in West London against racist murders. Shane got up and made a really good speech, and he was someone who'd never been involved in much political activism before. There he was, he was given a platform, and suddenly empowered. Shane, and I think everyone else, got a real buzz out of the empowerment for him there.

TOBY HOPKINS

West London became the sight of another action by OutRage! later in the year. The local MP, Harry Greenaway, had been reported as intimating that cottaging or cruising led to anti-gay violence, and that Michael Boothe had brought it on himself. Greenaway's lack of sympathy was judged homophobic, and an action was planned for a vigil outside his house, with £90 set aside by the group for the buying of 1000 candles and four torches for a demonstration on 19 October.

We all went over to Ealing Broadway and brought lots of candles with us – I had to carry the bloody things from the tube. We had an advance scout who pointed out which one was his car, and put the candles round his car to stop him running away. As if that's going to make a difference! He came out on the steps, and we all hissed him.

ADAM JEANES

In an informal capacity, David Allison from OutRage! attended Michael Boothe's funeral as a show of support. He was the only member of the group to do so.

And a day by the seaside

Shortly after the Michael Boothe march, the International Conference for the Family was organized as a front for a handful of right-wing and religious organizations to gather in Brighton to promote an agenda based on 'family values'. The conference boasted many high-profile personalities, including Diana, Princess of Wales, Valerie Riches of Family and Youth Concern, Mary Whitehouse, Digby Anderson of the Social Affairs Unit and a rumoured appearance by Mother Teresa of Calcutta. Former GLF member Martin Corbett had researched the make-up of the organizing group and discovered it had links all over the world with right-wing moral crusaders, which were not being publicly advertised. In an historic and daring escapade, Brighton activists took to the stage as Princess Diana was speaking to make a peaceful protest with placards saying 'Lesbian Mothers Are Not Pretending'. The action attracted major TV and press coverage and at the OutRage! meeting that evening, 12 July, the action was commended.

Nevertheless, OutRage! planned its own action against the Conference for the Family the following Sunday, 15 July. The main focus of the event was to protest against moves by David Wilshire to amend the Embryology Bill so that agencies offering Artificial Insemination by Donor would have to take into account a child's need for a father. An OutRage! press release stated 'We demand the right of access to safe donor insemination through clinics. We demand the right of women to control their own bodies, to decide when, and if and how many children they will have.'

A double-decker bus had been booked for an OutRage! day out at the seaside, with two major actions planned; one would take place inside the Brighton Centre during the conference, while another group of protestors would conduct a noisy demonstration outside. The intention was to disrupt a speech by Otto von Hapsburg, the pretender to the Austrian throne.

Our hacking of it came very much from OLGA, who had been following the right-wing scene. There was much discussion about whether we'd fill a double-decker. The OutRage! zap was basically a picket. We stood outside the Conference Hall and there were lots of us screaming and chanting. That's where the great OutRage! chants began.

TOBY HOPKINS

I think the main usefulness of that demonstration was simply that people had a hugely entertaining time taking the piss out of the Christians.

KEITH ALCORN

There were leaflets being distributed calling for funding to be withdrawn from the Terrence Higgins Trust, leaflets calling for the age of consent for gay men to be raised to 25. We basically stood up in waves. I was on the outside, and every now and then these security staff, who were really young people, about 17 or 18 at most, dressed up in white – they looked like angels – just viciously threw people out. We were outside singing 'There's more of us inside!', like football fans, 'More inside, more inside, more inside!'

JOHN JACKSON

I was the only one who didn't get slung out, because I didn't do anything worth getting slung out for. I had bleached hair, so I was getting talked to and I told them all I was with that group out there, and they were quite supportive. The general feeling was that they were ripped off. They'd paid exorbitant amounts of money so that all these rich nasty shit-heads could have their free air tickets.

DAVE BUNNETT

Although outraged at the conference, many found themselves having fun on the double-decker to and from Brighton, treating it as much as a day trip as a protest. It was exactly that sense of fun and community – putting the camp back into campaigning – which OutRage! would continue to try to imbue its zaps with in the future.

NOTES

1 Figures quoted from 'Policing Without Prejudice' by Peter Tatchell, in *Gay Times*, September 1990, and research on gay murders by David Smith, which appeared in *Gay Times*, June 1990.
2 Michelangelo Signorle is a prominent American activist and journalist. See below, p. 63.
3 The term 'broad based group of lesbians and gay men' has since been amended to include queers and bisexuals.

THREE

Stolen Kisses, Parting Glances

It established itself almost immediately as being about street issues, street theatre to present gay and lesbian issues not just in the gay press, but cynically and specifically about manipulating straight media to counter the tide of homophobia we saw in the mainstream press.

CHRIS WOODS

They started with the belief that you could change the world by printing stories in newspapers.

DAVE BUNNETT

OutRage!'s high media profile, largely due to its own band of journalists within the group, was becoming its chief success and failure. OutRage! was beginning to challenge the media silence, and its hostility, to gay issues. As more media attention was focused on OutRage!, its members began to question what that media was for, and the direction that OutRage! should be taking. For those who understood how the media worked, it was perhaps easier than for those who were more naturally distrustful.

Meanwhile, OutRage! merrily continued embarrassing the Metropolitan Police by drawing attention to their victimization of gay men for consenting sexual behaviour. In particular, attention became focused on police arresting gay men for kissing in public, under eight different pieces of legislation which could be 'interpreted' by police officers, most notably Section 5 of the Public Order Act 1986 which had originally been introduced to curb football hooliganism and violent street riots.

A newspaper article said that there had been two people arrested, a couple of years before at a night bus stop, because they had been kissing each other – there could potentially have been an old lady near and she would have been upset, one imagined. It was as flimsy as that. I was a lawyer, so I went and looked it up. I remembered ACT UP had had things like 'Die-Ins', and that a fun and media-friendly way would be to have lots of people kissing each other. People were saying should we have it in the city, or Buckingham Palace, and I wanted to have it slap bang in the middle of London. There was Eros, the God of Love, and it seemed completely appropriate.

PATRICK McCANN

Patrick's idea snowballed, and the 'Kiss In' proposal became hugely popular within the group. Once plans had been finalized for the afternoon of 5 September 1990 OutRage! began publicizing it. At planning meetings, it was acknowledged that there might be a risk of arrest and that the police had already indicated they might have to take action 'to maintain order' under Section 14 of the Public Order Act. OutRage! agreed that they would not disperse if asked by the police, they would not refrain from kissing, but that legal observers and stewards would be on hand with cameras to protect participants from police action, possible homophobic attacks, and to prevent provocative or inappropriate demonstrations of affection. There was also a troop of cheerleaders to urge everyone on, and the first appearance in Britain of a new London House of the Sisters of Perpetual Indulgence.[1]

I remember being a steward, and Peter Tatchell was going around – as he always does, bless his heart – and he said 'I want you to go round and make sure they don't do anymore than just kiss!' I felt like the Sex Police!

JOHN JACKSON

We produced the leaflets for that. We got hold of the pictures from *Square Peg* – we had to sift through lots and lots of these pictures to find one we thought suitable. I remember [Peter Tatchell] criticizing the leaflet because it didn't say 'Printed & Published by OutRage!'

ADAM JEANES

It really captured gay imagination. By that stage, we knew there was going to be press. Even if there were arrests, that would just fuel the controversy. What we thought, and as it turned out correctly, was that they wouldn't dare.

CHRIS WOODS

We did liaise with the police in some detail. They tried to pen us into a triangle, and when they weren't going to accept that we were going to push that away, we had to announce to people to get out of the pen and surround the whole of Eros.

STEVE STANNARD

All these things are very simple. You say 'let's have a kiss-in', you produce a leaflet, you hand it around, you've got 50 or 60 people at a meeting, most of those are going to go along, most of them will bring their friends. It was well publicized in advance, it was in the centre of London, it couldn't fail.

DAVE BUNNETT

I'd never kissed my girlfriend in the street before, and it was so exciting being able to do that, people cheering and clapping. I suppose, because I've done a lot of work in the theatre, I liked the way they were using theatrical devices. I thought to myself, 'Oh, I can contribute to that sort of thing.' I started to go regularly after the Kiss-In.

LYNNE SUTCLIFFE

As soon as I got there there were a whole lot of people that I knew from the GLF days. The GLF demos I'd been on before, I'd been pretty much up on. But this was people shouting things, with banners, placards, arguing with people, arguing with the police. I thought, 'I don't think I want to be involved in that, thank you!'

JOHN BEESON

I remember the actor, Richard, climbing up Eros – the bloody thing swayed! And he did crack it, they had to repair it. Even the police said 'Bloody hell!'

LISA POWER

We knew at that point that we'd cracked it. We knew we'd discovered a formula for actions that would bring large numbers of people out, get people very excited, get huge amounts of press coverage and generate a debate about the issues we were campaigning on, not just making a spectacle of ourselves. It did also have an impact on people's confidence about being openly gay in the West End.

KEITH ALCORN

It established OutRage!'s profile. It was the moment that transformed OutRage!'s image from a ragtag group of activists into a glamorous and spectacular group who could stage these large-scale events.

EDWARD KING

The action had gone perfectly, with around 400 people turning up, and no arrests. Even a group of builders, who had been jeering the crowd, were told to stop by the police. Indeed, the assembled crowd began wolf-whistling them instead. The press attention was huge, although the *Guardian* ran a picture of the action with a caption 'Kiss Of Death?' and the *Independent* claimed that 'Unless homosexuals wish to alienate the public they should conduct themselves with restraint.'

After our own

Not everybody toed the OutRage! line on queer visibility and sexuality. Many had been so accustomed to anti-gay prejudice and homophobia that even 'gay' pubs and clubs became prone to OutRage! zaps. The first gay club to feel OutRage!'s wrath was the Paradise Club in Islington. At the meeting which discussed finalizing arrangements for the Kiss-In, a report about an attack on a man leaving the club was raised. He had been attacked at knife point and thrown against a shop window, with another helper hospitalized. Paradise had refused the men entrance back into the club, an echo of a similar alleged incident a couple of months previously.

The issue of anti-gay violence was given added impetus when a GALOP member was beaten up outside the Lesbian and Gay Centre as the meeting was being held, resulting in the Centre manager having to issue reassurances to customers that there wasn't a band of queerbashers outside the building. The group voted to zap the Paradise Club that night, and donned OutRage! T-shirts to leaflet the club and protest to the management.

I urged that. The Paradise was the first of a number of zaps where we were actually targeting the gay community itself, and people were freaked by this, they were not prepared for it. People were really angry with a so-called gay institution that was letting the side down.

CHRIS WOODS

It was a very good sign of what OutRage! could do. We entered into negotiation with the management, I went in to see the manager, to talk to him about what had actually happened. The community was frightened, reasonably frightened of street violence. The management was looking into it, and the bouncer got the sack in the end. It was an achievable goal.

SIMON WATNEY

The action forced a number of concessions from the management, including an apology for mistreatment of queerbashing victims, a promise to provide sanctuary for victims of any possible future attacks, the maintenance of video cameras to deter attacks, funding for a leaflet detailing potential dangers and the promise of future collaboration with other clubs to promote local safety. In addition, as a gesture of goodwill, the Paradise extended an open invitation for OutRage! to sell whistles, T-shirts and distribute leaflets.

However, the following year, two women attending an OutRage! meeting on 21 July claimed that they had been mishandled by the bouncers, and urged OutRage! to zap the club again. The week before, Paradise had held a fundraiser for the Lesbian and Gay Rights Coalition, which had been formed by OutRage!, and handed them a cheque for over £1000.

These two women had clearly been beaten, and claimed that this was by the bouncers from Paradise. It was almost all gay men there, two or three women, who were clearly disinclined to believe these women and I got really angry. I'd been present when men had walked in and made claims, and had been believed, but because it was two little dykes who were known to be drinkers, they were all going 'Sorry, we need more proof.' I stood up and made a stirring speech. It turned out not to be true, of course. I feel I was right about the principle, but wrong about the example.

LISA POWER

The zap resulted in a meeting with the Paradise management, who did carry out an investigation and discovered that the accused bouncers had not acted unfairly. OutRage! did later acknowledge that it had made a mistake.

Paradise wasn't the only club in OutRage!'s targets. The popular Brief Encounter, in the centre of the West End, was not only one of the most successful and profitable gay pubs, but also one of the most commercially viable bars owned by Bass Taverns in London at the time. There were, however, a number of reports that the pub manager had stopped same-sex customers kissing on several occasions.

Somebody had been kissing in the pub. The music had been turned off, and somebody had announced over the speakers 'That couple in the corner, stop kissing!'

ADAM JEANES

They'd had a long history of being harassed by the police themselves, and like many gay bars they'd often get involved in self-censorship just to allay the police.

STEVE STANNARD

OutRage! hand-delivered a letter on 20 September asking for the manager of Brief Encounter to give an explanation, demanding a response by 26 September. With no response, OutRage! visited Brief Encounter again on 28 September, handing out leaflets and warning that further action would take place. Following the success of the Eros Kiss-In as a blatant show of same-sex affection, OutRage! publicised a Kiss In at Brief Encounter on 10 October. Around 30 people attended, and were neither evicted nor told to stop.

We infiltrated the place and stickered it from top to bottom and blew whistles and kissed as the bouncers freaked out. That was possibly the most chaotic zap of all time, because the management – who were desperately trying to drown out the whistles – turned the music up and as the music went up, the whistles got louder, and so the music went up. All of these gay men with their beers just standing there with this totally fucked look on their face, like 'What is going on here!'

CHRIS WOODS

Although no specific undertaking was given, OutRage! did not zap Brief Encounter again for its 'no kissing' policy, and other bars also seemed to adopt a more proactive approach towards expressions of gay affection. Like the Paradise, Brief Encounter was zapped again the following year after its decision to hold a 'fish night', whereby gay men were encouraged to bring their women friends to the bar. On 9 July 1991, OutRage!'s anti-censorship focus group, PUSSY (Perverts Undermining State ScrutinY) organized a zap.

It was fun. When we walked in, these guys just ran out the back door. We got loads of flack from a few of the straight women who were in there. I'd always assumed, and having never been in and having heard great tales about the Brief Encounter, that it was a men-only bar, but there were straight women who said 'What the fuck do you think you're doing?' The manager got very, very angry with what we were doing and the only thing I regret about that was that we didn't actually get old fish to be taken in. That was the original plan, that we were going to go to the docks, get yesterday's catch and dump it all over their counter. There were probably more of us there than there were customers by the time these guys had run off or run downstairs.

MEGAN RADCLIFFE

Unknown to them, there was a dyke in the group called Anne Marie from America, and Tessa Boffin. They'd got together some rotten fish from Billingsgate market and dumped them behind the bar. They went 'Get these fish out of here', and they said 'You asked us to bring our fish along, we've brought our fish along. They like it here, they want to stay. We're going.' They had to shut the bar down because of the smell of the fish.

JAMES KIERNEY

They had planned to get loads of fish and they didn't. They got like two fish or something, which Anne Marie had inside her jacket and she'd had them all week to try and make them go off, kept on her radiator or something. I think kippers or something really smelly. There were cardboard fish as well, that had been made.

LYNNE SUTCLIFFE

I've worried about it since. I think it was right and proper to do the protest, but I don't think it was OutRage!'s place or brief to do that. It was another rite of passage – it was saying there's no one we can't shout at if we want to.

STEVE MAYES

We could have gone to a lot of bars with the same idea. Brief Encounter were wise enough to get free publicity out of it. They were just stupid enough to admit the fact to somebody who phoned up, and we righteously got very, very angry about it. Everybody knows that straight men call us fish. I've realized over the years that there are certain things you have to admit will happen on a daily basis. They had another fish night a few weeks later and where were we? Somewhere else!

MEGAN RADCLIFFE

In general, OutRage! had a very good relationship with the commercial gay scene, and major venues such as the Market Tavern, the City Apprentice and the Royal Oak held extremely successful and popular benefits for OutRage!, which major gay cabaret stars such as Adrella and Jeremy Joseph were keen to support.

Policing the PIG

On 16 August 1990, following on from the demonstrations at Hyde Park and Ealing, OutRage! took its protest against anti-gay police activity directly to New Scotland Yard with a noisy demonstration, demanding that the police take more action against gay bashing, change in how minor sexual offences are dealt with, and monitoring of anti-gay attacks.

I went down and somebody handed me a placard, the way these things happen, and of course there weren't very many women there so I got put in the front row.

LISA POWER

Very early on, I realized that if OutRage! was to have credibility and effectiveness it needed to be able to back up its extravagant, spectacular zaps with good research which identified very clearly the scale of discrimination and violence against lesbians and gay people. I devoted a lot of time to producing the fact sheets that went with OutRage! press releases. When we talked about queerbashing, gay murders, the facts were there, accurately presented and properly sourced. It proved that the claims by the government and police that they weren't targeting gay people were false. It even exposed the myth of liberalization that many people in the gay community had internalized and accepted.

PETER TATCHELL

About 25 people had attended a fairly traditional picket, but the police response had been dismissive. One police representative, Inspector Hubbard, left a radio interview with Peter Tatchell claiming she would not talk to him or any group he represented. OutRage! voted unanimously to support Peter and his actions, but had also been informed that Inspector Hubbard was already seeking a community meeting with up to 20 'bona fide' lesbian and gay organizations.

The Gay Business Association and helpline organization Friend had been involved in negotiations with the Metropolitan Police since 1987. Their most successful result was in Friend worker Matthew Windebank designing training packages on gay issues for the police. However, these closed negotiations didn't include the wider gay community and seemed ineffective in tackling broader issues. The Metropolitan Police claimed that it was difficult to liaise with the gay community because there was no one voice to speak to.

Together with GALOP, OutRage! drafted a letter in August 1990 which it sent out to 70 London-based lesbian and gay organizations, outlining a Lesbian and Gay Policing Initiative. At the same time, following Inspector Hubbard's suggestion, the Gay Business Association was having secret meetings and attempting to set up its own Policing Initiative. The GBA were keen to contact groups such as the Monday Group and Stonewall, but not OutRage! Through the intervention of Stonewall, a meeting was set up with the GBA to attempt to solve the problems which were occurring. OutRage!'s Policing Initiative Group (PIG) was clearly up and running and heading for a confrontation with the more secretive arrangements being made by the GBA.

At a meeting between OutRage!, Switchboard, GALOP, Stonewall and the GBA on 25 September, a draft Statement of Aims was agreed, ratified at a later meeting on 30 September. This stated that:

1. The LGPI is a broad-based, non-politically aligned coalition of London lesbian and gay groups.

2. It will provide a representative and democratic forum to discuss our concerns with regard to policing.

3. As an organisation it will aim to develop common strategies, and a collective voice for negotiations with the Metropolitan Police service and other relevant bodies. Its objective will be to establish more accountable and productive relationships between these organisations at both a local and London-wide level.

4. The LGPI will seek to establish lesbian and gay dignity, equality and safety before the law.

We felt that the provocative confrontation with the police needed to be backed up with credible, practical negotiation to get tangible reform that would get the police off our backs and get to work protecting queers instead of persecuting us. OutRage! collectively came up with the idea of establishing a lesbian and gay forum where all interested community groups could meet to thrash out the basic agenda and reform that we wanted. That led to the creation of the lesbian/gay policing initiative.

PETER TATCHELL

The Policing Initiative was my idea. *Capital Gay* was based in Camber House in Mount Pleasant and in the same building and on the floor below was GALOP, and I was always in and out of their offices. I talked at length with Philip Derbyshire. Ironically, even though I'd helped to set it up, I wasn't allowed to do anything with [LGPI] because I was a journalist and the Met wouldn't allow a journalist in.

CHRIS WOODS

There was an obvious agenda on the part of those who were journalists, who had their own agenda for OutRage! They were looking across the Atlantic, they wanted to see OutRage! develop into a propaganda organization, but which had doors open to it within authority, within the political hierarchy. I didn't discount the fact that it would be possible to bring pressure to bear on the police. For me, that was much more a question of we weren't going to accept their policies, for example the harassment of gay bars over supposed noise nuisance… instead of a pre-meeting to discuss what was going to be the focus of our intervention with the police, there was a discussion about how awful the *Pink Paper* was and what a pile of shit it was. I made it quite clear I was going to take no part in it.

STEVE STANNARD

The end result was a meeting between the Metropolitan Police and the Lesbian and Gay Policing Initiative on 2 October, which raised more controversy due to the behaviour of some OutRage! members.

I was presented, along with everyone else, with the decision of a small group of people. There was no binding nature between us. There was going to be a joint press conference and as far as I was concerned, they'd already decided who was going to present that, so I said I wasn't going to have anything to do with that.

STEVE STANNARD

[Steve] came along, and he wasn't expected to come along, he wasn't mandated to come along, he just turned up, and it would have been too humiliating to chuck him out. He left halfway through because we wouldn't let him do anything, he was just there as a wind-up. He was trying to pretend his pencil box was a tape recorder or something childish. I remember Martin Corbett turning up and saying he was from GLF Information Services, which had not actively existed for at least 15 years, and the police didn't know any different. Jackie Forster [was] saying we should walk into the meeting, refuse to answer any questions, then walk out again, and teach the police a lesson. We wanted a commissioner to come and talk to us, just on principle. I don't think we had anything we wanted to say to him – other groups want it, we want it!

LISA POWER

The Lesbian and Gay Policing Initiative continued to meet, and began to establish a rapport, however tentative, between the police and the gay community. In December, there was increased tension when the police raided the popular Coleherne bar in Earls Court, as customers were having a drink after a funeral. OutRage! organized a march from the pub to the Earls Court police station on 3 December and liaised with customers from the Coleherne to put pressure on the police, who eventually apologized and agreed to meet representatives of the local gay pubs in a local forum.

To continue the pressure, OutRage! organized a 'political march' of over 600 people, led by a large 'pink dragon' to the Winter Pride festival on 9 December. The march took as its slogan 'Police Protection, not Persecution' and started at Horseguards Avenue, going to Malet Street via New Scotland Yard. Four OutRage! members, two men and two women, delivered a letter addressed to the police Commissioner, Sir Peter Imbert. The letter had nine major demands, including making sexual orientation part of the Met's Equal Opportunities policy, disciplinary procedures for anti-gay remarks, the recruitment of lesbian and gay officers, a Community Liaison Officer, monitoring of anti-gay attacks and an undertaking to stop *agents provocateurs* at cruising sites.

We adopted a two-pronged strategy of both confrontation and negotiation. There was no let up in our direct action against police homophobia, but at the same time we did sit down and propose practical measures to eradicate discrimination. It was typical carrot and stick tactics. We found that the harder we attacked the police, the more we ridiculed them and exposed their homophobia, the more amenable they became to the proposals for reform.

PETER TATCHELL

Although it was controversial, I think that's one of the lasting achievements of OutRage!, because that directly led to lesbian and gay liaison officers within the Met. It opened the door that had previously been closed, by both sides, through mutual distrust. It took a lot of courage for a radical gay organization to trust the Police. There was a breakthrough meeting at the London Lesbian and Gay Centre where there were four senior officers who talked about policing of the gay community and for the first time they started to listen to us on cottaging.

CHRIS WOODS

The night of the long knives

By this time, OutRage! had four distinct Committee Groups – Actions, Fundraising, Media and Office – as well as its Finance Officers. The groups were due to make reports at the beginning of every meeting, with the main group then splitting up to discuss upcoming actions. There were concerns about the facilitation of meetings, and how and who would be chosen to speak. Although ostensibly democratic – everybody had a chance to speak at OutRage! meetings, and anybody who turned up had a vote – in practice, many felt that OutRage! was controlled by a handful of people, known informally as the Polit-Bureau. Moreover, the question of what fighting homophobia meant was bogging down general meetings. At times, OutRage! would support other organizations – such as Lesbians and Gays Support the Miners, who received a financial donation from OutRage! – and at other times OutRage! would insist that it was merely about directly challenging homophobia. There was suspicion of left-wing infiltration into the group, particularly from the Revolutionary Communist Party.

Because it didn't have a structure, it was you turn up, you speak, that militated against women getting involved. Stonewall, for all it was vilified, had institutionalized parity, and if you ran out of women, you stopped recruiting men. I used to get very frustrated with OutRage! because all these men would stand up and say how democratic OutRage! was, anyone could walk in and stand up and speak, and they didn't realize that the only people who did that were the people who had the confidence and had been trained that they had any right to stand up and speak. It was almost always white men, mostly middle class. It was a fucking intimidating atmosphere in these meetings at times. I was in tears once, and I'm pretty tough!

LISA POWER

It became almost thuggish, cheering and applauding people when they said things – it's very difficult to dissent from something somebody has said if 20 people are cheering and shouting. I tried to restructure meetings, to break up in small groups. There was one meeting where I successfully put that through. It was very successful; a group of women were able to sit around and found themselves talking at an OutRage! meeting for the first time.

DAVE BUNNETT

There was always this problem where new people turned up to the group and never came back. I appointed myself as The Welcoming Person.

You'd go down to the basement and there'd be all these hopeful little people arriving for OutRage! and I told them what it was all about. I'd never been in a meeting-led organization before – they were saying 'You are OutRage!, we don't have a membership.'

ADAM JEANES

There was a real core who effectively ran OutRage! in a very undemocratic way. It was a core of activists, people like myself, Keith Alcorn, Simon Watney, Linda Semple, Gillian Rodgerson, Jean Frazer, Shane Broomhall, David Hurlbert. All the big rifts in OutRage! came about from that lack of honesty. We were the ones doing things, and my honest belief is that in any democratic organization, there's always going to be a core of people doing things and they're the ones where the power really is because they control the agenda and the minutes.

CHRIS WOODS

I stood up at the end of [a] meeting and said 'Thank you very much for ending on time, but next time can you make sure you don't overlook democracy.' A lot of people were talking about the state of the meetings. William Lester introduced some man who wanted to discuss group therapy with us, how groups can become comfortable with each other. This man stood up and started discussing group dynamics and how he, as a focus, could help us overcome the problems.

ADAM JEANES

Where it got out of control was [when] people got rightly pissed off by the fact that there was this cabal. The shit really hit the fan in terms of the RCP [Revolutionary Communist Party]. There was a battle that went on using OutRage! people as fodder, which understandably upset an awful lot of people.

CHRIS WOODS

Tensions were mounting over the Policing Initiative, particularly revolving around Steve Stannard's presence in the group. He had been approached by a minor radio company to give an interview, but was banned from doing so, as he was not the agreed spokesperson. At the beginning of October 1990 a bizarre series of events led to underlying political tensions within the group coming to the fore.

There were some really dirty tactics going on. We were having a secret meeting at Simon Watney's one night to discuss how to deal with Steve

Stannard and his gang and Simon's answerphone went. It was Steve Stannard posing as a Sky journalist, trying to set Simon Watney up.

CHRIS WOOD

We played the message back and I said 'That's Steve Stannard's voice.' Everybody listened to it again. We suddenly realized what we were dealing with, the degree of bitterness that had sprung up in the group and the lengths which both sides were prepared to go to in order to deal with it.

KEITH ALCORN

I think it was Keith Alcorn, in a comment to a radio station, that perhaps the police should be patrolling cruising areas to protect gay men. I jokingly left a message on Simon Watney's answer machine purporting to be a North American reporter from Sky News. It was such a funny message, and I gave my own telephone number. Simon Watney couldn't have been under any illusion who left it.

STEVE STANNARD

Hello Mr Watney this is Sky Television. It's regarding an interview given on radio yesterday by Mr Keith Alcorn of Outrage!, we're having difficulty getting hold of him, but it's regarding the, we understand Outrage! are inviting the Metropolitan Police to patrol certain areas, certain parks and commons in London, er, where we understand attacks on gay men are taking place and areas that they use to arrange sexual relations. We would be very grateful if you could contact us. If you could ask for, er, Tyler Smith [End of Message]... Oh hello, this is Tyler again. The number you can reach me at is 081 533 **46. Thank you so much.

TRANSCRIPTION OF ANSWERPHONE MESSAGE

We knew something might be happening because Shane had said in the office 'Oh, we've got him now!' and it didn't register until the meeting on Thursday.

AJAY

I remember thinking at the meeting 'this is very big' and they'd packed the meeting with people who were pissed off with Steve Stannard. There was a big report-back from the Lesbian and Gay Policing Initiative, so we thought they were all there to hear what the report-back was. You could hear people were trying to get to the LGPI bit and there was a bit of shifting around and hurrying. Steve stood up after Shane had spoken, and he said the immortal line 'Thank you, Shane, for that very macho presentation.'... There was a phrase like 'He's a liability, or a security risk and we have some evidence to that effect.' Instantly, someone produced a cassette player with an answerphone tape in it. Keith Alcorn stood up and handed out a transcript of what the tape said. We were all just amazed. The tape was clearly Steve. He sat there, and I remember his words were 'This is a stitch up.' I left the meeting, I was furious. I stood up and shouted and handed my key over to David Bunnett, who got very upset. He said 'No, don't do that.' I had to go back, because I'd left my coat in the bloody meeting, on the chair in front of Simon Watney who, as I walked in, was standing saying 'I'm scared to leave this building tonight!', and he'd uttered the immortal line 'I'm probably the busiest gay man in this town!'

ADAM JEANES

People described it as the best theatre they'd seen in years. There were a lot of people there for the first time who said they thought it was the best night out they'd had in ages, and they kept coming back because of that.

KEITH ALCORN

Virtually all of the people who supported my position as treasurer left, as I did, and went upstairs. At least seven people I spoke to were under the impression I'd been involved in some sort of fraud. There was no question of that.

STEVE STANNARD

It was really filthy tactics, which is what politics can be like. I don't regret fighting for what I believed OutRage! was for. It was a really important point, that this was a gay organization that wasn't going to be dragged down by left factionalism. I guess we – the cabal that I was part of – won, but at a very appalling cost. I don't think OutRage! was the same after that. I lost my job as a direct consequence of that, I was sacked from *Capital Gay*.

CHRIS WOODS

Steve Stannard was a great asset to OutRage! He put in a huge amount of work and made a very important contribution to the group. He also made some mistakes but I think half the accusations against him had no basis in fact. Sure, he came into the group from a revolutionary background but I'm not aware of any attempt by him to manipulate OutRage! away from its core agenda, at least no more than dozens of other people have tried! If Steve was guilty of that, then there are probably dozens of others who were equally so. Steve did make a mistake but I would have preferred that he admitted that, that the group acknowledged his contribution, and forgave him, and that he had remained within OutRage!

PETER TATCHELL

The group was absolutely controlled by the gay mafia from Oxbridge. There were people who had a different view of where OutRage! should be going. To their eternal discredit, the gay mafia jumped on them and accused them of entryism, and a left-wing plot, which was so astonishingly far from the truth it really was a McCarthyite witch-hunt.

TOBY HOPKINS

The only people I knew of in OutRage! who were involved in any clearly defined politics were my co-treasurer, who remained as co-treasurer, who had long been associated with the RCP, quite openly!

STEVE STANNARD

This conflict kept festering for months and months but essentially what had happened was that we'd made it very clear that we weren't just going to give in, that the process of attrition to which groups like OutRage! were normally subjected wasn't going to work on this occasion and that OutRage! was just about lesbian and gay stuff.

KEITH ALCORN

Hark, the herald fairies shout

Steve Stannard was replaced by John McVeigh as co-treasurer, and a letter was sent to the bank emphasizing that Steve had not been removed for financial reasons. The result of Steve's removal was that a plan put forward by Dave Bunnett for a rolling programme of actions, culminating in a march on Winter Pride, was set back. The march itself happened, and OutRage! also had a stall at Winter Pride, a head-shaving event to raise funds, and also performed a Christmas Nativity on the cabaret stage. Having been in existence for only eight months, OutRage! was proving popular and populist, with a real place in the community it was claiming to serve. Neil Wallace initiated plans for a Christmas celebration of the Queer Family, which would be held in the centre of Covent Garden, where a large Christmas Tree played host to more 'traditional' Christmas events and carol singing. Rather grandiosely titled the 'Covent Garden Christmas Celebration for London's

Extended Family', the aim of the event was to 'combine politics and entertainment' with carols led by the Sisters of Perpetual Indulgence, Linda Semple's mum giving a speech, Jeremy Joseph leading a parlour game, a speaker on lesbian motherhood, drag queen Regina Fong's Hall of Homophobes and symbolic presents for the lesbian and gay community. There was a Bang Club benefit later that evening in Tottenham Court Road, with 250 free OutRage! tickets, 100 of which were distributed to homeless lesbians and gays.

The first thing I saw was the Family Christmas, which was very impressive. I found it very moving, very well attended. There was a minute's silence in honour of lesbian and gay teenagers who had died. We ended up singing 'We Are Family' and carols with the lyrics suitably altered.

FERNANDO GUASCH

Nobody seemed to remember the words to anything, we just sang 'na na na na'. That was another good thing about the early OutRage! actions, they were slightly chaotic, but it really didn't matter. It felt like we'd hijacked Christmas, which was great.

LISA POWER

Even as OutRage! was singing away for the Twelve Days of Christmas ('on the fifth day of Christmas, my true love brought for me – five cock rings!'), there were ominous moves within Parliament and the government against lesbians and gay men. By the end of December, its first year in existence, OutRage! was already beginning to organize around a 'Hat-trick of Hatred' of legal issues affecting both lesbians and gay men, and which would bring new impetus to OutRage!'s fight against homophobia as 1991 began to dawn.

NOTE

1. The Sisters of Perpetual Indulgence are an order of gay male nuns, whose main aim is the expiation of stigmatic guilt and the promulgation of universal joy, through habitual manifestation. They have chapters throughout the world, but started in the USA in the late 1970s.

FOUR

Queering the Pitch

Even as plans were underway for the Covent Garden Christmas celebration, the general meeting on Thursday 13 December 1990 was presented with information about Clause 25 of the Criminal Justice Bill and the Butler Amendment to the same bill. Clause 25 proposed tougher sentences for violent and sexual offenders. In particular, it referred to three consensual gay offences: soliciting and importuning; indecency between men, and procuring. The Butler Amendment, tabled by Tory MP Chris Butler, proposed a sentence of up to ten years for knowingly infecting another person with HIV.

Although the Butler Amendment was dropped, Clause 25 was a major attack on consensual gay sex. OutRage! quickly saw that a national reaction was needed, and one which could bring on board serious media discussion. A letter was drafted for a campaign targeting MPs, which incorporated five questions including demanding why the government lumped consensual homosexual acts with serious sex crimes such as indecent assault, incitement to incest, under-age sex, indecency towards children and indecent photographs of children. The letter ended by simply asking 'Will the government now take immediate steps to delete the three consensual homosexual offences (solicitation by a man, the procuration of homosexual acts, and indecency between men) from Clause 25 (1) of the Criminal Justice Bill?'

Clause 25 brought together strands of OutRage!'s earlier policies of fighting against homophobic legislation. Over 2500 men had been convicted or cautioned for the offences in 1988, the last year for which figures were available. Solicitation could be flirting, winking, smiling, chatting up or even exchanging phone numbers. Procuring of homosexual acts could mean anything that helped two men have sex, including letting out a spare room or introducing two men in a pub, even if they were over the legal age of consent of 21. Indecency between men could be any show of affection, including cottaging, kissing, hugging, holding hands. The proposal of Clause 25 was that these offences should be punished with up to five years of imprisonment, followed by five years of psychiatric supervision.

At the same time, in a new move to attack 'pretended' families, a proposed 'Paragraph 16' of guidelines issued by the Department of Health for the Children Act would prevent lesbians and gay men from fostering children. The guidelines claimed that

It would be wrong arbitrarily to exclude any particular groups of people from consideration [to become foster parents]. But the chosen way of life of some adults may mean that they would not be able to provide a suitable environment for the care and nurture of a child. No one has the 'right' to be a foster parent. 'Equal rights' and 'gay rights' have no place in fostering services.

The move came after Norman Tebbit had attacked a grant to the National Foster Care Association to organize a training on 'An Equal Service for Lesbians and Gay People' and after two local authorities, Waltham Forest and Newcastle, had been attacked for allowing lesbians and gays to foster and adopt children.

Then, on 19 December 1990, a long-awaited verdict from Judge Rant on 11 gay men arrested after a police operation against sadomasochism was another blow against sexual freedom. Operation Spanner was the result of a police investigation begun in 1987, after police believed videos of SM sex showed a man being murdered. In fact, none of the injuries depicted in the video required medical attention. Not only were the men given sentences ranging from fines of £2000, but some were given up to four years' imprisonment, as the judge rejected 'consent' as a legitimate defence. The implication of the ruling was that any mark left from a heavy love bite, or any form of body piercing, that is for anything other than 'decorative purposes', may be illegal.

When the 'Hat-trick of Hatred' was discussed in January 1991, OutRage! began to mobilize for a larger organization to coordinate a campaign, resulting in a major mass demonstration and rally. To launch a community response, OutRage! invited organizations and individuals to a meeting on 13 January 1991 at the third-floor meeting room of the Lesbian and Gay Centre. The meeting attracted lesbian and gay organizations as well as leftist organizations. The meeting took the decision that the campaign should be run by lesbians and gays themselves, under the title banner of 'The Lesbian and Gay Rights Coalition', with the main focus of the work being building for the national demonstration and march on 16 February.

The Coalition for Lesbian and Gay Rights was basically a stooge organization, it was a complete fake. We set it up so we could manipulate the triple campaign. It was basically a way of dealing with Ajay, who was always moaning on at us about getting the wider community involved. When the campaign's over, we'll pull the plug on the organization, so OutRage! doesn't have to get its hands dirty. What actually happened was we pulled the plug on it and the water didn't actually go down, it kind of lingered on for a couple of years as this irritating non-organization.

CHRIS WOODS

The first meeting I went to was when they had stuff in the gay press that week on Clause 25. I went at a very exciting time, with people getting really worked up. For me personally, it was tremendously important because it was the first time I had come across happy gay people. I'd come across rather sad, self-hating people who were marginalized in the SWP [Socialist Workers' Party]. There was a big argument about whether straight people could come and we in the SWP had to argue tooth and nail that straight people should be allowed in, which I'm very embarrassed about. I think there was a strategic alliance with the Sisters of Perpetual Indulgence, the oppositionists in OutRage!

SIMON EDGE

I was there from Stonewall, and someone who had always been important to Stonewall but never turned up – and had never been seen in public – was a guy called Douglas Slater, who was Secretary to the Leader of the House of Lords, and very instrumental in founding Stonewall. [He] couldn't say boo to a goose, because he was our inside man in Parliament. He turned up to this meeting dressed head to toe in leather, stood it for about 20 minutes and said 'Good God! Is this what lesbian and gay politics is all about! I'm going to have a beer!'

LISA POWER

It was a cynical attempt by us to kick-start gay/lesbian politics back into radicalism. What OutRage! was trying to say was that they were on a par with Section 28, which they weren't. It was a useful way of bringing OutRage! and other organizations on-side with Spanner. To link up Spanner with those two other issues made it more difficult to attack Spanner. Spanner was the clearest case of show-time homophobia that Britain had seen in the last 30 years.

CHRIS WOODS

Get up, get out, get even!

As the Coalition prepared for its mass demo, OutRage! began planning its own zaps and demos about the proposed homophobic legislation. The first action was a scrubbing of Parliament, to clean it of its homophobia, on 17 January, coinciding with the new spring session of Parliament.

I'd come out in the July. I went on the Pride march of that year, felt the power, realized that if I belonged to this community I ought to give something back to it. I'd never heard of OutRage! at that time, looked in *Time Out* and saw there was something called a Coalition. [I] went to one of the Coalition meetings and then I felt I wanted to know more, to do more. On the Thursday morning the following week, I was outside the Houses of Parliament with a scrubbing brush in my hand. It was a side door and very quickly the police pushed us on, but the deed was done and the photograph was in the papers. Then we went to Downing Street.

BETH LANE

In a similar demonstration, for a day of action called by the International Lesbian and Gay Association, on 14 February, OutRage! attempted to 'scrub the Union Jack clean' of homophobia. With the Gulf War on, it was deemed too sensitive to burn it. Around 30 people and media cameras turned up, and similar actions were carried out in New York, San Francisco, Sydney, Athens, Amsterdam, Copenhagen, The Hague, York, Southampton, Aberystwyth, Edinburgh, Newcastle and Manchester.

A more daring action was planned for 6 February. Bow Street Police Station, the site where Oscar Wilde had been taken a hundred years previously, became the site of a mass turn-in of 'sex criminals' who would dare the police to arrest them for procuring, soliciting, or under-age sex. Although tongue-in-cheek, the action technically put the participants at risk of investigation and arrest, if the police were willing to take it that far. Derek Jarman, who had held a benefit screening of his film *The Garden* a few days before, volunteered to turn himself in, and pop star Jimmy Somerville also lent his support.

Around 500 people turned up, despite the freezing cold and a blizzard, although the weather made a glorious backdrop. Lining both sides of the road next to the Royal Opera House, protestors held placards including slogans such as 'I'm guilty because he's handsome', 'How big is your bigotry?' and shouting chants including 'We're here, we're queer, and we're not going to the opera!', while a portable stereo blared out 'Sex Crime' by Eurythmics.

It got a lot of attention from the press. It had been formulated in such a way that it was very much a participatory event, as all the best OutRage! events were. The thing I remember best was there were loads of people on the other side of the road underneath the Royal Opera House. Someone complained to the manager about all these people clogging the pavement up, and his response was to put the awning out to keep the snow off the demonstrators.

KEITH ALCORN

People were standing outside demanding that the police arrest them! I don't think even GLF ever did that. And, at the end of the day, not a single prosecution. Individuals were vulnerable, but as an organization it seemed the police had taken some sort of tactical decision that it would do more damage to arrest us than it would not to.

CHRIS WOODS

They were confessing to the most ludicrous offences, it was a complete mockery. A lot of the best OutRage! actions were concerned with mocking the powers that be. The turn-out was phenomenal. We got many more people than we expected. Even if people didn't go, they were still talking about it.

KEITH ALCORN

I was quivering, I'd never done any public speaking on that level at all. I can't remember what I finished with, it was something really controversial 'cause it said the word 'fuck' – 'Keep your laws off our fucking bodies' – or something like that, and stormed off!

ALAN JARMAN

I was gobsmacked at the power of the event. The street was lined with all these queers making a noise. The police just did not know what to do. I immediately latched onto this opportunity to have fun, cause mayhem and do something useful along the way. I didn't see very much, couples going in and kissing on the steps, but it was incredibly low key. At that stage I saw myself as an observer. I adopted this role of watching and monitoring. It was an incredibly intimidating group, but having a camera, which was a skill that nobody else had in the group, was a way of validating my presence and held me in there in times when I would otherwise have disappeared.

STEVE MAYES

The Coalition Mass Demonstration took place on 16 February, with around 10,000 people attending a march through London, finishing at a rally in Hyde Park. OutRage! 'hijacked' Eros at Trafalgar Square to do 'mildly naughty things' as a repeat of their infamous kiss-in. Speakers included MP Ken Livingstone, Peter Tatchell, Christine Moss, a lesbian mother facing deportation to Australia as an illegal immigrant, Alex Owolade from the Lesbian and Gay Campaign Against Racism and Fascism, and OutRage! members Neil Wallace and Charles Anglin who 'confessed' to under-age sex. One woman was arrested for foul and abusive language after chanting 'Two, Four, Six, Eight, Is that copper really straight?' She was released later.

One of the happiest moments of revenge in my life: we were on the march and for some reason Alex [Owolade] was a steward, which is so unlike Alex it's not true. I'd done several stints at demonstrations where Alex and Alex's friends had bullied people mercilessly, and I just wound him up. I behaved atrociously, and he kept saying 'Move back! Move back!' I turned round to Alex and said 'What's the matter, Alex? Are you doing what the police want?' Alex used to say that to me, and I was using every line that he ever used on me, and he was so furious because he was chief steward and he couldn't do anything about it. I remember hearing Peter Tatchell giggling hysterically behind me while I was doing it.

LISA POWER

That evening a 'Valentine Queer Love Shock Rave', with appearances by John Hegley, Regina Fong, and others, raised over £1000 for the Coalition. It was held at the Paradise Club, less than a week before OutRage! zapped it for a second time. A later demonstration in Manchester, the Liberation demo on 13 April, had up to 20,000 attending a carnival-like protest against Clause 25. The Coalition itself, originally set up solely for the February mass demo, continued to meet for a number of months, although numbers were severely diminished and it became little more than a mouthpiece for left-wing sectarianism. It held a last gasp open meeting on 24 November but, dogged by alleged financial irregularities and in-fighting, failed to continue in any meaningful way after that.

OutRage! carried out another demonstration against Paragraph 16, but after much discussion it wasn't getting enough attention because it was seen to be a lesbian issue. It took place on Good Friday, 29 March. Around 30 people demonstrated outside the Department of Health. The demo was low-key, but a highlight was a dyke bus-driver blowing the horn and waving as she passed by.

Eventually, the guidelines for Paragraph 16 were made more neutral, and significant concessions on Clause 25 were won. The Spanner ruling went to appeal. The following year, OutRage! held a Spank-In at the High Court in the Strand, with around 40 people turning up, with judge's robes, leather, whips and stocks. *Capital Gay* reported that the 'police only started twitching when one enthusiast appeared to be trying to fist-fuck a Sister of Perpetual Indulgence'.[1]

At the time, I was working for Angus Hamilton. It was obvious that this was a hugely important case and that we should be marking it. That was the first time I'd organized anything. Most of the demonstrations were prompted by an individual who had a particular interest, and then that person would say here's why, this is what we do. I'd looked at the case, about child exploitation, complete nonsense.

ROB KEMP

The looks on people's faces as they walked past was my distinct memory. It didn't seem like anybody knew why we were there, they weren't looking at the placards, they weren't looking at the leaflets because they were too busy staring at people smacking each other. That was also empowering, somebody doing that sort of thing in front of an hour or so of traffic and all the people going past, who'd probably never seen anything like it in their life. I felt like 'You know now, and you know that I'm not going to sit down and have you smack me around with your laws.' It wasn't extremely well attended, mainly because it was cold.

MEGAN RADCLIFFE

It's a queer world

Even as the Coalition was putting OutRage!'s in-your-face style on the national agenda, and OutRage! groups were starting up in Manchester, Liverpool, Coventry, Hull and Scotland (often centred around colleges and universities), the new style of 'queer politics' was attracting more and more attention, both within the gay press and mainstream media. Queer Nation in America had been vocal and powerful, challenging not only homophobic mainstream society but also the more conservative and stale 'gay rights movement'. Those OutRage! members who had been to the States and worked with Queer Nation saw the potential to influence OutRage! even more, structurally and ideologically.

I'd gone home [to San Francisco] for a Christmas holiday, and I attended a couple of Queer Nation meetings. This was at the height of their creativity, power and influence. There were hundreds of people at the meetings. The organization had grown so large that it could only function through specialized committees, but it wasn't bureaucratic. The committees all had cool names, the members seemed to have fun. I realized that if OutRage! kept growing, we'd have to begin doing something similar in order to function efficiently.

DAVE HURLBERT

There were so many things going on within OutRage!, and so many things people wanted to do, it seemed a great idea to break things down into smaller cells with different names and different functions. I remember there being some opposition, and I remember Peter [Tatchell] saying he thought the cell structure began to undermine OutRage! as an organization because the whole was sometimes less than the parts. The big meetings favoured pompous speakers and they disinclined those who may not feel competent to speak, but often had the most interesting things to say. The cell structure empowered those people within the smaller groups, on subjects they decided they were interested in. Those groups were basically responsible for themselves, they'd go out and get their own publicity, do their own stuff – there were sometimes four, five OutRage! actions going on in a week.

CHRIS WOODS

It was just another adoption from America, but the principle was good, which was that it encompassed everybody, but it became very elitist. It was promoted by a small group of people who were postmodern journalists or academics. It felt like they were apostles of queer. It promoted some more strong dykes getting involved in mixed stuff for a while, that was a good aspect of it.

LISA POWER

Queer politics was a new politics. It was post lesbian and gay, but was very different, very exciting. It was Queer Nationalism. It was represented as just about a word, but there was a generational struggle going on, which was akin to the struggle between 'homosexual' and 'gay' in the early seventies. To me, sexuality is in a state of flux, it's a changing thing, a metamorphosing thing. Gay, which had been a radical, revolutionary concept in the early seventies, had become this conservative, strained value system in the nineties, which commercial organizations had a vested interest in maintaining. Queer became a proxy battleground for the real battle, which was about identity, who had the right to call themselves what.

CHRIS WOODS

I still think the queer thing is ghastly. It's either very childish and embarrassing or it's reclaiming language, which is fine as far as it goes. I think there was an elitism going on, Chris Woods's own view, who thought it was body piercing mainly, and setting themselves apart from queens at Bang. It was people saying we're not just happy-sexy-shag-a-lot gay people, but you also have to be sexy, shag-a-lot, angry, militant gay people.

SIMON EDGE

It's like saying there were only two camps – you could be gay or you could be queer. I don't think that's the case. Most people identify with a gay lifestyle, and for many women who've had affairs with their next-door neighbours, they'd never think of calling themselves lesbian. When *Gay Times* did their special issue [on Queer], they didn't have a single article by a lesbian. We were excluded.

MEGAN RADCLIFFE

The decision to adopt a structure which was more closely aligned with Queer Nation's – that of having 'cells' – was taken in January 1991, to allow for more actions to take place. This also led to a restructuring – or more accurately, renaming – of existing groups. The fundraising group became QUID, finance became the more endearing QUANGO (Queer Accountants Never Go Out). Following Queer Nation's lead, more outrageous acronyms became popular within OutRage! The prize for the most convoluted must surely go to a group which attempted to present an anti-censorship festival at the South Bank, but ultimately failed after no one could agree on a common working definition of fighting censorship. The group's acronym became SHAGPILES – Screaming Homos Against Gutless Prissy Icky Lawmakers Enforcing Selibacy (*sic*)!

With the new names came changes to the meeting. As well as a facilitator elected at each meeting, new roles were adopted; a 'timekeeper' was responsible for keeping debates within agreed time limits (usually anyone who had a watch) and two 'vibewatchers' were responsible for assessing the 'feel' of the group, and trying to diffuse tension. In reality, the role of the vibewatchers became increasingly controversial, as vibewatchers were often able to manipulate the feel or direction of a meeting.

There were very clear tensions within OutRage! itself over the word 'queer'. Although many arguments were put forward to justify the word – including the ideas that words needed to be reclaimed, to take the power of the word away from oppressors, and the notion that 'queer' could collapse many different identities (lesbian, gay, bisexual, black, white) under the rainbow flag of 'outsider/different' – many still felt uncomfortable. In OutRage! *queer* was seen as sexy, challenging, a form of radical chic that encapsulated OutRage!'s ideology of self-organization within the gay community. For some, however, it echoed the way language was used against lesbians and gay men and, in particular, the way that the tabloids denigrated lesbians and gays with words such as 'poofs' and 'lezzies'.

The debate in OutRage! came to a head when Chris White, feeling that OutRage! itself was acting oppressively by using the word 'queer', distributed flyers in a meeting threatening to burn himself as a symbol of the oppression OutRage! was carrying out.

> Everyone reached for a light, which was one of the cruellest things I ever saw in OutRage!
>
> **CHRIS WOODS**

A heated argument ensued, with accusations of blackmail, emotional manipulation, and bullying, ending in a compromise to give more scope for discussion of the issues involved. OutRage! called and publicized a public meeting on the use of the word 'queer', held at the Lesbian and Gay Centre on 17 March. Cordially, the meeting agreed that people should respect the rights of individuals to self-define, and use whatever labels they felt appropriate, and that sensibilities should be respected. Although the meeting closed amicably, the same splits reappeared over coming months, with a series of vitriolic letters in the gay press, and eventually the formation of an unofficial 'alternative' OutRage! called 'InRage', set up by Chris White, which made occasional appearances at OutRage! demos.

'Cliff Gay Jibe Fury'

Even as the debates about queer continued, extravagantly 'queer' film director Derek Jarman was taking more than a passing interest in OutRage!, and supported the group not only with fundraising events, but also with personal appearances at demos and pledges of support for the group.

> He was just amazing and the only prominent person to give OutRage! any support. Everybody else considered it to be too dangerous and that to me says a lot about where Derek's politics were. He got OutRage! immediately and gave it a lot in terms of ideas. It was of a piece with Derek's character, which was that he was always prepared to nurture new talent. He always had huge amounts of time for people who had new ideas and an interesting take on the world and that's why he saw OutRage! as something which he really wanted to help. Derek was always very clever at reflecting the spirit of the times. He knew that OutRage! was the place where the energy was during that period.
>
> **KEITH ALCORN**

In early 1991, Derek Jarman was at Bray studios in Windsor filming a queer version of Marlowe's *Edward II*, the story of a queer king's battle against his backbiting landowners, and his love for a young but unpopular man. Jarman's version drew a strong analogy with modern Britain, its homophobia and systems of power. He invited OutRage! and the Sisters of Perpetual Indulgence to take part in the filming for a day, as supporters of the Queer King Edward.

A group of about 20 OutRage! members were hired as extras. We were in a section of the film which spliced the real story of Edward II's homophobic murder with real-life queer activism against anti-gay violence.

PETER TATCHELL

I was working as a cook in the police. They didn't know anything about anything. I wanted a day off for filming, it was important, so of course they wanted to know why I wanted the day off. When I explained, they said 'You're not allowed to belong to other organizations when you're in the police without telling us.' I said 'I didn't belong when I first joined the police.' I was very quickly asked to leave, so I did.

I well remember the first bit, which they didn't put in the film. They had us in twos running round wooden steps.

BETH LANE

OutRage! are here for the day, sound drums and trumpets! Peter Tatchell looks after them like a hen with chicks, I rush about as we never have had so many people in a day, 90, and our resources for looking after them are stretched, and we all want it to be a 'good day'.

DEREK JARMAN[2]

During the lunchtime break, quite by accident, some members of OutRage! discovered that Cliff Richard was in an adjoining studio doing a sound recording. Gathering together a posse they barnstormed their way into the studio and disrupted the recording session with cries of 'Come out Cliff'. There were scenes of chaos and uproar as the session ground to a halt and security people tried to shield Cliff Richard. It was all over in a couple of minutes but left a lasting impression with reports in some of the papers the next day about Cliff Richard being confronted with reports about his sexuality.

PETER TATCHELL

More than 30 gays dressed as nuns and priests stormed a rehearsal studio where the 50 year-old bachelor boy was practising for a charity tour. The gays... blew trumpets and waved placards. They tried to break down the rehearsal room door and chanted 'Come out of the closet, Cliff, and declare yourself a full blown homosexual.'

THE SUN[3]

The incident made the front page of all the tabloids the next day, and for a while it seemed that the film *Edward II* might be in jeopardy if legal action were brought. However, the film was produced, Cliff Richard got to deny that he was gay, and OutRage! made the movies.

Speaking out of turn

The National Viewers' and Listeners' Association (NVLA) had long battled against representations of homosexuality on screen, and were arguing forcefully against the screening of programmes such as *Oranges Are Not the Only Fruit*. Led by Mary Whitehouse, they were effective in forwarding conservative views on censorship of television and radio, even though numerically they represented a tiny proportion of the viewing population. Censorship was an issue of much interest to OutRage! at the time. Jenny White was being prosecuted for having imported lesbian sex videos from a San Francisco feminist erotica store. Customs had seized the material and prosecuted under the Customs Consolidation Act 1876, which had also been used to justify raids on gay bookshops such as Gay's the Word and West and Wilde. OutRage! took a longer-term interest in the Jenny White trial, and picketed the court throughout the hearing in April, which she eventually lost.

OutRage! was tipped off that the National Viewers' and Listeners' Association would be holding its AGM at the RAF Club on 23 March, when MP Kenneth Baker would be addressing the group. OutRage! applied to the NVLA for further details, under a private address in Leytonstone. The aim was to have a demonstration outside with placards and speakers, while OutRage! members in straight drag attempted to infiltrate the meeting and disrupt it.

We were so sure that there would be incredibly tight security. We were all really, really nervous. We turned up with our suits on. I remember the guy at the door said 'Where have you come from?' I said I'd seen it advertised in my church and he asked me where it was, and I said 'Balham.' He said, 'Oh, I live in Balham. Do you know St Michael's'? I looked a bit blank, and he said 'It's the Catholic Church' and I went into a bit of a panic. We signed our names on the register and sat down.

GRAHAM KNIGHT

It was one of the first things I did. Dave Hurlbert was my 'brother', we got in first. I had to sign and I wore my RAF badge because it was in the RAF Association.

BETH LANE

Kenneth Baker stood up and said there'd been a lot of people demonstrating in the United States, and at that point someone from OutRage! got up and said 'There's a demonstration here as well.' And we just ran riot, blowing whistles, running around. It was Mary Whitehouse's anniversary as well.

GRAHAM KNIGHT

About ten minutes into Mary Whitehouse's speech, everybody started shouting and screaming and videos were going and we soon got ejected. I lost the badge, [I was] thrown down the steps.

BETH LANE

I was deeply impressed when I realized one could occupy space against the wishes of the people. That was a very revealing moment. The audacity of it was impressive. That was the first time I came across [photo-journalist] colleagues professionally as well. It was my own political outing.

STEVE MAYES

The action had been simple but effective. As OutRage! had gone in with video cameras, posing as press, everything had been recorded to boot. A further zap occurred as Kenneth Baker made an escape in his car, only to be swamped by OutRage!, and needing police support to get away. OutRage! had contributed almost a third of the people at the meeting and confirmed in their own minds how small and insignificant the NVLA was.[4]

Wedding belles

It wasn't all doom and gloom. OutRage! wanted to have fun, celebrate the queer family. What better way to do it than have a Queer Wedding? In June, invitations were sent out to the gay community to attend the wedding of the year in Trafalgar Square, between 6.00 and 8.00 p.m. on 12 June to celebrate not only long-standing relationships, but also one-night stands, friendships, sex-friendships, threesomes, S&M relationships. The invite promised 'Music, Dancing, Dementia, Love Rites, Wedding Cakes, Queer Guest Stars Galore!' with 'Wedding attire suggested, as well as Radical Drag, Leather, Feathers, Chains, Urban Glamour'. As well as an opportunity for some real fun, OutRage! were aiming to publicize the ways in which queer couples were discriminated against, including denial of custody, adoption, immigration, inheritance and tenancy rights.

In the first Dutch queer wedding, two lesbian activists, Janna van de Hoef and Pauly van der Wildt, were married on 5 June 1991 at Deventer civic hall. On the eve of the Queer Wedding, Theresa Gorman had introduced her Cohabitation (Contract Enforcement) Bill into the House of Commons, aimed at giving legal recognition to co-habitees, which would have included lesbian and gay partnerships. As a 'Ten Minute Rule' bill, it had no chance of making its way into legislation, but provided a focus for discussion of lesbian and gay partnerships before the law which could feed into OutRage!'s street theatre.

On the day, 11 same-sex couples pledged vows, dressed in wedding dresses, morning suits, drag, leather and rubber. The vows included 'I promise to love and adore you and spend the rest of my life with you', 'I promise to share my Body Shop kiwi fruit lip balm with you', and 'We promise to love and spank each other for the rest of our lives'. Songs included 'Going to the Chapel' and 'I Am What I Am'. Instead of traditional presents, gifts of free British citizenship, the right to adopt children, tax benefits and inheritance rights were given. The rights were theatrically snatched away by a 'judge' saying 'These presents are only for boy–girl couples. Normal, God-fearing straight people! We don't allow presents like these for lesbos and poofters' to boos from the crowd. The view was echoed in real life by one man who objected saying 'I am queer, but I don't go along with this performance. It makes a mockery of gay relationships.'[5] He went on to shout that he hated women and would kill them and removed his false teeth, snapping them at bystanders and claiming he had AIDS and would bite them to death. The police were called as a scuffle broke out. On stage, a wedding fairy burst out of the 'wedding cake' throwing confetti and shouting 'Love! Light! Happiness for queers everywhere... some day those presents are going to be available for all of us, no matter who we are and who we love', presenting new gifts of guts, pride and freedom from hetero hell to enable the couples to cope in the meantime.

I was going out with Sarah at the time, but she didn't feel brave enough to marry me, so I married Hannah. I remember thinking about the actual rights that were going to be involved, and were going to be written on paper plates and thrown out into the crowd. I liked the way that some of the service was real and moving because some of the couples were real and serious. I remember Patrick and Lofty marrying, and promising not to scratch their Madonna records. [Julie] married a life-size cut-out of kd lang. I knew it would be quite a media sexy action. I was aware of the passers-by. I remember feeling quite safe because the group in the Square that was supporting us was definitely in the majority.

LYNNE SUTCLIFFE

I felt it was not the politics that OutRage! should be playing with. OutRage! sometimes veered too much towards assimilationist politics… I was upset at that action.

CHRIS WOODS

I was very concerned about the Child Support Act, which was coming in, and seemed a clear State definition of what a couple should be. It was clearly the State saying women had to be married to men if they had babies – it seemed to me that this was a very important message which should be addressed at the Queer Wedding.

TOBY HOPKINS

We went off to The Bell, and they'd given us a wedding cake, and we were really celebrating for an action well done. The energy from a successful action carried into meetings for weeks.

LYNNE SUTCLIFFE

FROCS Away

During 1991, one of the major arguments surrounding the new queer politics centred on 'outing' public figures as gay or bisexual. Outing had already happened in the States, where demonstrations by ACT UP had publicly named officials known to be gay, claiming that their sexuality should be public knowledge. Queer Nation took this further, articulating strong arguments for outing gay men and lesbians in positions of influence or power. *Outweek*, a radical queer publication, regularly outed major figures, and many of its contributors – Gabriel Rosetti, Michelangelo Signorile – claimed that sexuality should be a matter of public record, and that many 'straight' publications deliberately hid or 'bearded' gay public figures, even when their sexuality was important to a story being run.[6]

A major campaign using the label *Absolutely Queer* outing public figures on posters in public places took America by storm, involving pictures of celebrities such as Jodie Foster, Tom Selleck, Mel Gibson, John Travolta and Whitney Houston. The campaign dominated discussion of gay issues, and in particular representation of gay men and lesbians in the media. Inevitably, the discussion about outing hit OutRage!

Gabriel Rosetti, who was Editor of *Outweek*, wrote a brilliant philosophical justification of those situations when outing was permissible. It ruled out anyone other than people in positions of authority who were 1) denying their homosexuality while being known active homosexuals, 2) using their position of power to oppress other homosexuals and

3) enjoying the privilege of homosexuality at the same time. I was European Editor of *The Advocate* and we did three outing covers – Pete Williams, who was Assistant Secretary of State for Defence, a Governor in Florida and the third was some religious minister. I was involved in 'ethical outing' whereas in this country it seemed to be 'Well, we don't like him, and somebody said he was, so let's do it.'

CHRIS WOODS

I hadn't been out very long at all. I wasn't really out to my mother [but] doing national actions, and shouting and being very loud and also doing my play about coming out, *Fifty Ways to Tell Your Mother*. I remember being really troubled by the idea of outing, probably because I wasn't that out myself, and the idea of somebody outing me was really scary. I remember really arguing for the fact that we should have no official policy on outing.

LYNNE SUTCLIFFE

Because we couldn't come to a consensus, the OutRage! general meeting voted to have no policy on outing.

PETER TATCHELL

It was the classic OutRage! compromise – this is the organization view, and anybody who wants to do anything different, clear off into a corner.

LISA POWER

OutRage! decided that it would not even have a policy on outing, because the issues divided the group absolutely down the middle. That decision led to some people getting together to look at ways in which outing might be used as a political tool.

Shane was doing my garden, so he used to be in and out of here. He was forever asking me which MPs were gay, and I realized I was having my brains picked so I kept fairly shtum. My attitude then was very anti-outing. I knew he was collecting names, and I knew they were going to do an outing campaign. I said 'I don't agree with you, but I'd rather know about it.'

LISA POWER

In early 1991, a set of posters featuring the pop and soap opera star Jason Donovan appeared in the West End of London. The posters showed an image of Donovan wearing a T-shirt with the words 'Queer as Fuck' superimposed on it. Jason was appearing at the Palladium Theatre in *Joseph and the Amazing Technicolor Dreamcoat* and the posters immediately spotlighted him. When the fashion magazine *The Face* reprinted the poster with an article about Donovan, he issued a writ against them. The original posters were later attributed to the outing group FROCS, which wasn't entirely accurate.

I remember Lofty coming into the OutRage! office one day and showing me this poster and he'd made fifty copies, and he was saying 'Do you fancy coming out and putting them up?' I was just laughing at him and saying it was completely pointless, and I really didn't want to be involved – not on ethical reasons, I just thought it was childish and puerile. Lofty put it up on a whim, not as part of any great political message. I remember looking at it and thinking that the poster was naff because it was a naff posture and he'd used Gothic writing for the *Queer as Fuck*. Little did we know that he would put these things up in exactly the right places and appear in *The Face*.

PATRICK McCANN

The posters inspired an appetite for outing amongst activists and also in the press. It was clear that outing was a media story, and that the media were interested in why, when and – most importantly – who would be outed by the gay community.

At one OutRage! meeting, I remember Peter [Tatchell] coming up to me. My view at the time [was] that people irrespective of political affiliation should be outed. I felt that anybody who was in the public eye, there was a duty for them to be out and if they weren't going to be out, I in a radical way was going to out them. Peggy said did I want to become involved, and this was definitely happening. I think Shane had already met with a *Sunday Times* journalist, representing this huge amorphous group FROCS.

PATRICK McCANN

About a week before the FROCS story hit the headlines I was approached by a journalist from the *Sunday Times* who had somehow got hold of the story that an underground gay group was about to out 200 top people in public life. That was the first I'd heard of it, although there had been whispers and rumours in OutRage! circles for some weeks previous. I was contacted by Shane Broomhall, one of the FROCS conspirators, seeking my advice on how to handle the media. He very cleverly realized that by keeping the identity of FROCS a secret, it would give them an element of protection against possible legal action and also add a conspiratorial flavour which would feed the media frenzy. Although I didn't agree with what FROCS were doing, I did believe there were legitimate political and ethical arguments in favour of outing. I thought it was right those arguments should be heard. I could see that the political effect of outing 200 leading public figures would be enormous. It would be a political earthquake that would demolish the existing structures of public debate around homosexuals in public life.

PETER TATCHELL

I think we claimed we had several dozen if not several hundred members, but in fact it was me, Shane, Dave Hurlbert and Lofty. Lofty had a flatmate called Matthew French. Matt came up with a name. Matthew wasn't involved in the group, didn't want to be involved in the group, because he didn't believe in outing. I'm not sure it's a name I would have thought of because Faggots Rooting Out Closeted Sexuality I didn't feel was an image that we wanted. We didn't necessarily want to associate ourselves with dresses, particularly as apart from Lofty I don't think any of us would really wear dresses in a big way. Also, the fact that it was only faggots in the title left the lesbian element out, but again that's because we were rushing.

PATRICK McCANN

On 28 July the front page of the *Sunday Times* carried an article titled 'Gays threaten to "out" MPs in poster campaign', in which FROCS were alleged to be making posters to out 200 prominent figures, including 52 MPs, 8 judges and 12 senior church figures. The article led to a flurry of phone calls from other interested reporters and all of a sudden FROCS was snowballing.

I didn't really know what was going to happen. I just knew that we were going to out people. I remember I was starting to make enquiries as discreetly as I could at work about where we could get pictures of MPs. We hadn't met to discuss this and what we would do. We just had this rough idea that we would out people. Peggy [Peter Tatchell] had asked me would it be all right for my phone number to be given out, to speak to journalists. Naïvely, I had said yes. Because there were so few of us, we decided we had to have one representative, but because there were in fact two of us who would be speaking we decided we had to have the same fictitious name. The name we took was 'Mikey Angel', a bastardization of Michelangelo Signorile's . We *were* going to out people, naïve as it may seem. My phone was ringing off the hook.

PATRICK McCANN

I began to feel some suspicion when FROCS were unwilling to talk about who they intended to out. Since I'd proven in my go-between work that I was totally trustworthy and reliable, I found it a bit surprising that they were reluctant to talk in more detail. I put down my suspicions to my own fondness for precision, detail and forward planning. During this period some reporters, particularly from the *Daily Mail*, began to close in on the people from FROCS. We all had a sense that we were under surveillance. There were always reporters lurking outside my flat in cars.

PETER TATCHELL

Shortly after I got all these phone calls, things started happening with my phone and I started getting calls from Shane. He was talking in coded language and it was clear to me that there was a suspicion that we were either being tapped or being traced. You just heard a clicking sound, and whether or not that's the sound of someone tapping I don't know. Shane was finding reporters on his doorstep. We certainly had people sitting in a car opposite for a couple of days. I was in a bit of a difficult situation because, funnily enough, I wasn't completely out at work. That, of course, made it difficult for me ethically. If I did the outing thing, I wanted to do it openly. Lofty came to pick me up from work one day and I had to stand in a doorway and he would walk past and if it was safe he would do something like touch his ear and I could then follow him and if it wasn't [safe] he would carry on walking... it was all very *Carry On Spying*.

PATRICK McCANN

The tabloids were unequivocally critical of the threat to out, and the *Sun* even published an article by out gay radio personality Paul Gambaccini condemning FROCS. In the few days that the FROCS saga hit the headlines, 'Mikey Angel' and his cohorts were condemned not only by the mainstream press, but also by gay groups such as Stonewall. In one incident, just before going on a Radio 4 interview with 'Mikey Angel', a Stonewall spokesman fed him the name of a gay MP – and then went on air to denounce outing. The *Guardian* carried intelligent arguments for and against outing, with a printed head-to-head between Derek Jarman and Malcolm Sutherland arguing that 'outing is a sign that the gay movement has come of age', while the General Secretary of Liberty, Andrew Puddephatt, argued that outing infringed civil liberties.[7] In probably the most reasoned article of the season, Neil McKenna in the *Independent* argued that outing, right or wrong, was the natural symptom of a homophobic country:

Outing is just another symptom of homophobic oppression; it is a high-risk strategy that will win few friends and will almost certainly make many enemies. That gay men and lesbians are prepared to consider using it at all signifies the desperation they feel at their lot... outing, paradoxically inspired by and feeding off the prurient interest of the media, will continue and escalate – a classic case of as ye sow, so shall ye reap.[8]

As the press pressure increased, the four FROCS members and their 'press liaison', Peter Tatchell, had to quickly think about the situation they were finding themselves in. Not only did they have to answer the questions about who they would out, they also had to decide who was to be involved in FROCS and how they were going to manage the media hysteria. The group had various discussions about 'widening' the scope of FROCS to include more people but felt unable to do so, for personal and strategic reasons. Instead, FROCS came up with an entirely new strategy, and hastily arranged a meeting in the utmost secrecy.

I remember Shane ringing me up and saying 'We will meet in that place near that place that is very cold' and it turned out it was the Prince of Wales pub in Coldharbour Lane near The Fridge in Brixton. We met at the pub, and I was walking towards it and this bicycle appeared with this man in a yellow macintosh with a yellow sou'wester. I heard this 'Pssst!', looked up and it was Peggy under the sou'wester. Peggy goes 'Follow Me' and I'm trying not to laugh and take it all seriously, and he cycles a little way up the road and then veers off into this little alleyway so I carry on walking and hear this 'Pssst! Come in here!'

PATRICK McCANN

By this stage we suspected that the threat to out 200 of the most senior officials was bound to attract the attention of the Special Branch and the security services. Our last meeting was in the stairwell of a block of flats off Brixton Road, at which point I was given new directions to go to another flat about three-quarters of a mile away in the other half of Brixton. Late into the night we thrashed out a plan to hold a press conference at the London Lesbian and Gay Centre.

PETER TATCHELL

Dave's idea was that we would say that the whole thing had been a hoax. We would hold a press conference and claim that we were going to out people, to which everyone would (and did) come and we would then say 'It was all a hoax, we only did this to show how homophobic the press was' and that would be great, it would let us off the hook. I was pretty angry and upset. I didn't feel that the benefit that would come to us by exposing the British press as homophobic was sufficient for us to lose a pretty valuable opportunity. I still think there would have been other ways to do it and that we were forced into that situation, which I felt was basically a cop-out. I remember going round to Malcolm's later in Camberwell and crying.

PATRICK McCANN

The press conference was called at the Lesbian and Gay Centre for Friday 31 July. The room it was held in was next to the OutRage! office, which had to be covered up for secrecy. The conference was packed with journalists from TV, radio and the newspapers. Lofty and Shane had been designated to read out a prepared press statement, which was handed around to the journalists.

They were absolutely convinced that we were going to out these people. They were on their mobile phones ready, they had their editors waiting, they had their phone calls open to the Houses of Parliament, so there was a complete buzz. I don't think we had their attention for very long before the press release told them that they weren't going to get anything. It was maybe one or two lines before Shane said the whole FROCS episode was a hoax, we never were going to out anyone. As soon as it became clear that it was a hoax, there was an audible groan. Some of the press who wanted to show their disfavour were already dismantling cameras as the press conference was going on... Lofty had to read out 'phenomenon' and couldn't do it and was completely petrified. I remember him saying something like '...and the whole press phenomenonon... phemonemanonn... phenomen... phenoman... *sensation...*' It showed that he didn't write it because he wouldn't write a word he couldn't pronounce. They'd dressed up for the occasion. Shane was looking very butch in chains and stuff, dark glasses, loving the attention. We were pretending we were very cynical... if that had been our intention at the beginning, that would have been fine, it would have been an OK thing to have done.

PATRICK McCANN

To an extent, the plan worked. The press were exposed as hypocritical – denouncing outing while clamouring for the names of prominent gay people so that they could publish them, and in some cases feeding names to the FROCS spokesmen. The 'outing' got lesbian and gay activism discussed in a way that had not been discussed before. Lesbian and gay issues had dominated the headlines for the week, and discussion had included not only outing but the place of lesbians and gay men in society, and their rights and responsibilities. At the following OutRage! meeting, even though FROCS was not technically anything to do with OutRage! itself, a heated debate ensued.

I was kind of kept out of FROCS because I was gay press and they thought that was a problem. It caused a lot of friction in OutRage! because it wasn't an official OutRage! thing, and yet it was always read that way. There wasn't a great sophistication on the debate on outing in Britain.

CHRIS WOODS

I was naïve at the time, the party line was against outing. I remember assuming everyone else would be against outing too. I was standing up at an OutRage! meeting saying I'd heard awful things that people were threatening to do outing and it was awful, we must stand firm against it, and realizing that 70 per cent of people in the room were in favour of it.

SIMON EDGE

I didn't feel that FROCS had a case to answer with OutRage! because we'd divorced ourselves from OutRage! The fact that some of us happened to be members of OutRage! did not make us answerable to OutRage! Nonetheless I felt an obligation to FROCS the organization, to Shane, to Peggy, to Dave, to Lofty, to fight the FROCS line and basically lie. I didn't feel that bad about it because I felt that a lot of the anger came across because there was jealousy. It's the typical British way – not to do anything and when somebody does something just to complain about it. We were being told we had thrown away this golden opportunity, and how other people were just about to do something on outing the next day. People had had 18 months, two years to get used to the idea and if they had wanted to do something on outing they would have. I don't think we'd have been able to go to OutRage! and say maybe we did fuck up. I don't think there was enough support in that room for us to say that. A lot of the people making the accusations never got off their arses anyway. Whatever we did must have done something and that was good. Although the opportunity was thrown away on that occasion, the next day you could have had up posters. You could still out people today. The issue was still there, is still there.

PATRICK McCANN

FROCS was over and done with in less than a week. It had dramatically opened up the arguments about outing in Britain, and polarized the gay community on whether it was a good tactic or not. Nobody had foreseen the amount of press interest, the anger and scale of response to outing. No one had been outed, but outing itself was a story. Underlining that story was the fact that OutRage! and the press knew there were closeted gay men and women in high positions who kept their sexuality a secret. If FROCS achieved only one thing, it was the recognition that queers were everywhere, and that the majority of people were happy to keep that little secret. It was not the last time that the spectre of outing would land OutRage! in hot water.

We just felt that the pressure was on and we needed to get out. That was a symptom or a result of our unpreparedness. Had we prepared we'd have done the calls off a mobile phone, we wouldn't have been traced, we would have had more people on board, we would have got our photographers lined up, we would have got our press releases lined up, we would have had press statements. Shane and I were giving interviews not knowing what the other person was saying. We would have had a single spokesperson, as opposed to two of us, one with a New Zealand accent, one with a camp English accent! I don't think it's a bad thing to say someone is gay. I don't have a problem with that. I think someone's sexual orientation is more or less a matter of public record, it's like someone is black or left-handed. It's a descriptive statement. If someone has chosen to give another image of themselves, then I think that's their choice.

PATRICK McCANN

NOTES

1 'Court spank-in', *Capital Gay*, 3 April 1992.
2 Derek Jarman, *Queer Edward II* (BFI, 1992), p. 122.
3 '30 gays in taunt at Cliff', the *Sun*, 12 March 1991. In fact, I was on the outing, which wasn't really an outing at all. Derek came up to the Sisters, and told us that Cliff Richard was recording in a hanger nearby. He told me it would make a great photo opportunity, and was well aware of what we might do. I went round telling the lads. We'd been told that Cliff refused to do charity concerts for AIDS (at that time – he has done them since) so we were thinking of doing a zap to confront him about that. Some of the guys went to do a reccy, found where Cliff was, but 'fell into' the rehearsal, not thinking that the door would be open. Once there, we had to do something, so we mumbled something, which attracted the security. It was almost a case of, someone sneezed and suddenly we were in Cliff's rehearsal and doing an action. I can remember shouting something like 'Why won't you do concerts for people with AIDS?' For the rest of the day, we were shunted around and escorted by the production company, and treated like schoolkids. We were given a dressing down, although Derek was supportive (well, he had to be really, it was his idea!). Interestingly, as none of us could get to a phone, there's always been a mystery as to who tipped off the media. Cliff's agent?

4 I went into the NVLA meeting with a nun's habit on underneath my coat. I remember starting to giggle as I wandered round the foyer, because it was full of people from OutRage! pretending not to know each other, who were also trying not to giggle. I remember Craig Moroney talking to one of the organizers. Craig had a strong Australian accent, and was pretending to be interested in a similar organization back home. Of course, the man he was speaking to had many contacts over there… We started off by clapping very loudly to anything any of the speakers said. We clapped loudest and longest, but not so much that it was suspicious. I was in the middle of a row of seats when the first zap occurred. I was preparing to go to the toilet to change into the nun's habit, but with the brouhaha going on, I became immediately obvious. After shouting my bit, I walked out, but most of the others were 'escorted' by very red-faced assistants. I changed into my habit outside in the end.
5 Reported in the *London Evening Standard*, 13 June 1991.
6 For a fuller account of outing and reasons for it, see Michelangelo Signorile, *Queer in America: Sex, the Media, and the Closets of Power* (Abacus, 1994).
7 'A helpful shove off the straight and narrow/ Private lives and public oppression', the *Guardian*, 31 July 1991.
8 Neil McKenna, 'Outing's bitter truths', the *Independent*, 29 July 1991.

FIVE

The Whores and the Three-Legged Man

Outing and the new queer politics aside, more local problems beset queer Britain. Increasingly, anger against many homophobic major British institutions was being highlighted in the Thursday meetings. Media coverage of gay issues often highlighted more general homophobic attitudes and practices within larger organizations. The Metropolitan Police had been targeted as a symbol of a homophobic legislative system and as discriminatory agents themselves. A new and equally significant target for OutRage! became the Church of England, in what was to become the start of an ongoing campaign against religious homophobia.

Following the new Queer Nation theory that things get done a whole lot better and quicker when you have an affinity group to do the work, a preliminary meeting of the Whores of Babylon on 24 February 1991 identified two main goals :

1. To campaign against the promotion of hatred and violence by religious organizations against homosexuals.

2. To stop the silent support of homophobia by religious organizations and to force them to take a stand on issues of importance to the gay community.

The Whores committed themselves to fighting homophobic behaviour and statements (not religious beliefs) and would not get into protracted theological arguments. The Whores of Babylon agreed that they would take on all religious institutions, but their first target would be the Church of England, as the most prominent religious group in the UK.

From the beginning of OutRage!, I'd tried to get other people worked up about this, but there wasn't much interest. I guess the Church of England seemed beneath contempt. But not for me. I knew a number of closeted gay priests, really evil creatures who hated other gay men almost as much as themselves. And I was sensitive to the damage being done. By condemning homosexuality the church was giving fagbashers a moral seal of approval. Martin and Aamir signed right up.

DAVE HURLBERT

The first target was immediately obvious: the enthronement of Dr George Carey as the 103rd Archbishop of Canterbury. Although Carey was touted as ostensibly liberal because of his support for the ordination of women priests, when asked 'Is practising homosexuality a scandal?' had replied 'Yes it is.'[1] On 12 March, the Whores of Babylon wrote a familiar letter to 'George' asking him to lay out the Church of England's position on homosexuality, on 63 murders of gay men since 1986, on homophobia, and particularly on teenage lesbian and gay suicides. The letter ended by demanding that the new Archbishop provide more positive pronouncements on gay issues:

You must state publicly that the church condemns all violence whether physical or psychological against gays and lesbians. And you must stop providing ammunition for anti-gay bigots by your pronouncements.

Dr Carey's response not being forthcoming, the Whores of Babylon planned an event to coincide with the Archbishop's enthronement at Canterbury. Working with gay groups in Canterbury, the Whores planned events with around 60 protestors to effect a high-profile zap.

I wrote a script, got the parts cast – the whole thing involved the burning of gay and lesbian martyrs. The intention was to perform this right outside the cathedral just as the religious ceremony began. We chartered a bus and loaded it with about 25 OutRage! members.

DAVE HURLBERT

I remember sitting at the back and we were all having 'confessions', terrible confessions, how many people had failed to have safer sex.

TOBY HOPKINS

The fundamentalists were there, and they were against George Carey as well. Alan Beck produced a leaflet outlining the history of Canterbury, so it was quite educational!

GRAHAM KNIGHT

The Canterbury police were there in plain clothes and uniform, and every time someone went off to the toilet, they would be followed by the police. They were very concerned – what we had planned for the day was just to walk round with Shane carrying a cross. The police had been expecting us to be what we had promised to be, which was a direct action group. I don't think we ever were a direct action group, we were a media action group and we were very good at it.

TOBY HOPKINS

We staged a protest at the gates to the Cathedral compound, couldn't get any closer than that because security was so tight. We shouted, whistled, chanted, danced and sang, much to the consternation of the police who were videotaping us from an upper window in the small plaza. Desmond Tutu passed by, smiled and waved to us. In fact, a lot of the arriving dignitaries seemed pleased to see us. After about an hour or so of carrying on, we staged our performance. The climax was our 'archbishop' flaying a group of lesbians and gay men with a bull whip, then burning these martyrs at stakes.

DAVE HURLBERT

The action was very successful, although there were allegations that the East Kent constabulary had arranged a hoax bomb scare to get the Archbishop out of the Cathedral. The following Sunday, 21 April, the Whores of Babylon also confronted a parish priest, Reverend Lister, at his parish church in Stepney Green, over homophobic remarks he printed in his parish magazine.

Preparations soon began for another large-scale event, but much more proactive in attempting to use the Church's own language and symbolism against itself. The adverts for 'The Exorcism of Lambeth Palace', the Archbishop of Canterbury's London residence, promised an event that would entertain as well as make political points:

GASP! as the Church has its homophobia purged out! CHEER! as the Archbishop repents his bigoted ways! Support your local psychosexual priests and priestesses as they exorcise and expunge the Church of hatred of homosexuals. All Sex Gods and Goddesses of Desire welcome… Help us rid the Church of prejudice. This could be the end of religious victimisation as we know it!

Elaborate plans were made for the Exorcism, and a full script prepared. The ceremony took place on Wednesday, 7 August, starting at 6.30 p.m.

We met on a big grassy lawn opposite Lambeth Palace. Lynne and Martin were on a stage and I was part of the religious band. We had finger cymbals and tambourines. People had joss sticks and we made sounds. There was a person who had a cue card. He was slightly draggy and he brought them on, and they said 'boo' or 'cheer' .

GRAHAM KNIGHT

There was a script and I learned the script off by heart so I could perform it properly. Martin Girvin was all gold. That was one of the first actions that Sarah came on with me. She dressed up with Mark Harriott as Adam and Eve. All she was wearing was an apple round her bottom and a tiny little bikini and she looked very, very sexy. The outfit that I was supposed to be wearing that day Mark Harriott had made me, and wasn't finished and I had to be sewn into it on the way there. I could hardly breathe. The head-dress was made of a coat-hanger and it kept getting caught on things. The sash I was wearing was a real priest's sash and I didn't know that until about half past three. I said 'Oh, that's a nice sash, where did the sash come from?' and it was like 'Oh. I think it's a real priest's one.'

LYNNE SUTCLIFFE

There was a general intro saying why we were there and what the church had done to us. The first thing was to purify ourselves, so we lit the joss sticks and the people on stage would say how many of us grew up in families of intolerance, how many of us had been queerbashed... if this is you, put your hands up and scream. It went through all the crimes of the Church, and we said 'We forgive you' afterwards, and then a minute's silence to remember our own experiences of being hated by the Church. We summoned the Demon of Homophobia to come up and the Demon of Homophobia was supposed to go in this effigy, made I think by Shane, all twigs and thorns and stuff, and we threw it into the sea, into the Thames. It was supposed to be torn apart, but it was just sticks and things. Then we handed out flowers to everyone at the end. I don't know what they were supposed to represent.

GRAHAM KNIGHT

The burning of the martyrs wasn't really very convincing. It was a nice idea, but just didn't work. The imagination of the action appealed to me, the ability to take an absolutely rock solid piece of the Establishment and turn it upside down. The assertion of our sexuality over the history and strength of the Church was a tremendously empowering experience. Just seeing that happen was a click in my mind that one could not only stamp and shout and throw your fists around, but you could adopt a position that was so strong in its complete inversion of society's views. The exorcism was a coming out for OutRage!, that real confidence of saying 'We are right – fuck off! The world looks different from this end of the telescope and this is what it looks like.'

STEVE MAYES

It didn't get the vast numbers we were expecting. It was a theatre piece really. It was seeing what worked and what didn't work.

GRAHAM KNIGHT

It was a slightly confused point, it didn't have the clarity of later events. Quite why Aamir was dressed in this strange Catalonian cum Ku Klux Klan garb defeated me at the time, and doesn't really make much sense, but [it had] a very strong presence. It was much more of a party, really. We were mildly stropzy in a minor sort of a way. It was a shame that it was raining, that it was very cold. 'A small exorcism in Lambeth, not many hurt' kind of thing.

STEVE MAYES

The Exorcism highlighted the Church's attitude to homosexuality, condemning 'homosexual genital acts' in the Higton debate during a Church Synod in 1987 and suppressing the Osborne Report, which was later revealed to encourage liberal change within the Church. The press enjoyed reporting Mark Harriott's comment that 'If Adam had found another Adam in the Garden of Eden there would be no homophobia in the Church and everybody would be so happy.'

Toward the end of the year, OutRage! was informed of a group called 'Living Waters' who claimed that, through belief in Jesus Christ, homosexuals could be 'cured' of their homosexuality, and had set up groups in America as part of the 'ex-gay' movement.[2] Although other groups in Britain claimed that they could also 'cure' homosexuality, the Living Waters ministry provided a target for three main reasons. First, they had recently published a book by ex-gay Andrew Comiskey which was being distributed in Britain, *Pursuing Sexual Wholeness – How Jesus Heals the Homosexual*. Second, the Living Waters ministry was founding a base for the group in Belgravia, at a church called St Michael's, under the direction of the Reverend Christopher Guinness. Finally, the group was about to fly over American ministers to oversee the founding and expansion of the 'counselling' service.

The Whores of Babylon sprang back to life at the prospect of such a marvellous target. The original idea was to enter the church and disrupt the service, but only those parts which came before the sermon so as to minimize offence to the churchgoers while still making an unequivocal statement. The first demonstration against St Michael's took place on 17 November.

St Michael's became a hobby, really. We discovered that Guinness, an arch-homophobe, was due to make his first appearance at his new parish church.

STEVE MAYES

We were sitting there singing. I'm like 'Oh my god, oh my god, oh my god, I don't know any of these hymns.' I felt that I really stuck out like a sore thumb. The four or five of us who went in must have stuck out. They must have known. I had all these eyes in the back of my head! It was fun, but it was frightening at the same time.

MEGAN RADCLIFFE

We duly dragged up in Christian drag and went in as members of the congregation, with our placards, cameras, whistles, all the things we needed to make trouble. As Guinness stood up to speak, Martin Harrington got up and shuffled to the end of the pew and very calmly walked up to the front of the church. Harrington took the microphone and just said 'Do not be alarmed.' At which point, the whole place erupted into total panic. 'Do not be alarmed. We are here to… blah blah blah.' A number of people who had been planted in the congregation duly whipped out their placards and also walked up to the front and formed a line across the altar rail, holding up their placards. My role was to take pictures.

STEVE MAYES

It was awful because of the reaction of these Christians, who screamed at us. We got thrown out of the church, which is an odd feeling. I'm not religious, but to get thrown out of a church seems a bit of a sap.

MEGAN RADCLIFFE

There was a lot of pushing and shoving and hitting along the way. Guinness subsequently came out to talk to us. 'Do come for tea, we'd like to talk to you about this.'

STEVE MAYES

The demonstration attracted a lot of publicity, not only from the gay press, but also from the mainstream and religious press. The British Association of Counsellors 'expressed concern' at the techniques used by the Living Waters group, and a member of the congregation left St Michael's and sent an anonymous donation of £50 to OutRage! in support of the action. Reverend Guinness agreed to meet for tea and sympathy, but nothing was ultimately achieved by the meeting. The demonstrations became weekly events, becoming more confrontational. A controversial leaflet was drawn up and delivered to all the houses in the area:

Queers Are Not Sick! Cure Heterosexual Hate! The latest outrage from the Church of England. Now they claim they can cure homosexuality! CAN THEY BOLLOCKS!

The confrontations were mostly good-natured, but on 11 December, both the police and OutRage! stepped up their positions.

We were inside the church. There was a christening going on, and the police had warned us they could arrest us under the Ecclesiastical Powers Act of 1836. We got in the *Church Times*, which was fun – 'children cried, old people left distressed'. We got into a lot of conversations with the parishioners. One of them was gay, and stopped going to the church.

FERNANDO GUASCH

[Guinness] wasn't a full-time member of the church, he was a visitor. A lot of the local people supported us, but they didn't like our style of demo. It worked – we got a lot of people on our side from that church. I remember a certain Sister [of Perpetual Indulgence] blessing me as I was led away in the back of a black Maria.

NICK CAVE

Although the demonstrations didn't stop the group meeting immediately, pressure was brought to bear on Reverend Guinness and Living Waters. For the first time, attention was drawn to the ex-gay movement, with the new Archbishop of Canterbury himself expressing concern at the movement. BBC's *Heart of the Matter* highlighted the issue, and the Lesbian and Gay Christian Movement launched its own enquiry into such counsellors. The issue of homosexuality and the Church became the next big thing after the ordination of women.

While the demonstrations against St Michael's Church were running, OutRage! zapped a Church of England press conference at the launch of its document *Issues in Human Sexuality* on 3 December. The document stated that clergy 'cannot claim the liberty to enter into sexually active homophile relationships'. OutRage! demonstrators unfurled banners saying 'Stop crucifying queers' and shouted down the bishops holding the conference, claiming they were responsible for queerbashing on the streets.

Although the Whores of Babylon effectively stopped acting as a group after 1991, their impact on OutRage! was enormous – both in terms of their ability to form and carry through actions as an affinity group, and in their influence on OutRage!'s policy on tackling religious homophobia. OutRage! became more hard-line on anti-gay religious oppression, and the campaigns subsequently became more intense, and personal.

Two fingers to the Three Legs

The Isle of Man, self-governing but a Crown dependency, had the dubious honour of being the only place in Western Europe where consensual homosexual acts were illegal, with buggery punishable by a jail sentence up to life imprisonment. Britain, having signed up to the European Convention on Human Rights, and having authority over the Isle of Man's foreign policy, had committed it to decriminalizing homosexuality. Despite this, the Isle of Man's own parliament – the Tynwald – had voted against changing the laws twice in the previous five years.

By spring 1991, things had come to a head. In February two deaths related to the police implementation of the anti-gay laws had drawn attention to the plight of gay men on the Isle of Man. The previous year, 21 gay men had been arrested and charged with gross indecency in a public lavatory close to the police headquarters in the island's capital, Douglas. A 35-year-old man, Kevin McCauley, was found dead in his car in early February, having committed suicide shortly after appearing in court for gross indecency. The same week, a straight man, Darren Wild, shot himself as police arrived to question him about his relationships with gay men. Although police claimed that they had only wanted to interview Darren about a motoring offence, gay activist Alan Shea claimed that the police had persistently harassed Wild about his support for gay men.

The publicity around the two suicides, and pressure from Alan Shea, brought the Isle of Man to the attention of OutRage! in February, and planning began for a series of actions. The Tinwald was due to discuss changing the laws, and OutRage! began a high-profile campaign to embarrass both the Tynwald itself and Westminster, whom they wanted to pressurize the Tynwald. OutRage! began by encouraging a letter writing campaign to the Home Secretary Kenneth Baker. In March, the Tynwald voted against changing the law and in April another controversial police campaign resulted in 12 men being sentenced for consensual homosexual acts, after police had 'persuaded' two men to reveal names and addresses to them.

The Isle of Man was planning to hold a stall at a large shipping exhibition being held at the Barbican Centre in London in May. An action was planned, and involved the controversial slogan 'Isle of Wanx', adopting a 'Flag of Shame', adapting the Isle of Man's three-legged flag, and highlighting the claim that 'The Isle of Man is bad business.' On 21 May, members of the group met dressed in 'business drag' at 9.30 a.m. at the Lesbian and Gay

Centre, just round the corner from where the 'Expoship 91' exhibition was being held.

I had to go as a Brazilian. Somehow, we'd got all these false cards and I'd got to use this false name to go in. I had to ask all these pertinent questions about shipping, but I really didn't know what I was talking about. I got left with the shipping [stall] and Peter [Tatchell] went off with another group around the back. We all came back for the final demonstration with placards.

BETH LANE

We disrupted it quite effectively. We stood by the stand, and shouted what they were, and made a speech.

TOBY HOPKINS

The protest hijacked the Isle of Man's self-publicity. As part of the continuing campaign, Isle of Man gay activist Alan Shea attended an OutRage! meeting in June to talk at length about the situation in the Isle of Man. OutRage! took a decision to take its protest to the Tynwald itself, planning a trip to the annual open-air meeting of the parliament in July. Shea, representing the Manx gay rights group Ellan Vannin, was due to hand in a petition for redress of grievance at the Tynwald's refusal to reform the Manx laws. OutRage! organized subsidized places to send members in support, and also arranged for six people to hand in a protest letter to the Prime Minister at 10 Downing Street.

On 5 July, dressed as a concentration camp victim, Shea ran the gauntlet of hissing soldiers and booing onlookers to deliver his protest. As he did so, OutRage! onlookers silently unfurled banners proclaiming 'We're queer, we're proud, get used to it', 'Legalise gay sex' and 'Queer today, queer tomorrow, queer forever'.

We went up to Liverpool, over on the ferry, spent the first night discussing tactics until about five in the morning and making placards. I ended up shouting at everyone, ranging from the Parliamentarians to little old ladies. There was a little man from the Church, a homophobic church stall with a booklet that was produced about how bad it was and what a sin it was. That was another ding-dong battle.

BETH LANE

The church stall, staffed by Christian evangelicals led by Mel Cheetham, became the target of an impromptu kiss-in as four couples kissed and were moved on by the police who told them 'not to push it anymore'. Onlookers shouted 'You want castrating' and 'They should be rolled down Slieau Whallian in a spiked barrel.'

We went back the next day. Someone said to me 'How brave you are to come.' I said, 'No it's not bravery, it's politics.'

BETH LANE

The following year, Londoner Michael Cole went on hunger strike to protest against the government's refusal to take action against the Isle of Man. Eventually, in April 1992, the House of Keys did vote to change the law, decriminalizing sex between men over the age of 21. Almost certainly the decision had less to do with civil liberties than the fear that the British government would intervene and the Isle of Man might lose its status as a tax haven.

Cruising around

Attacks on gay men at cruising grounds were still an everyday occurrence, and as an extension of the whistle patrols, OutRage! tried to 'outreach' them. Its first attempt was at a performance of the play *Teatrolley* by Homo Promos Theatre Group, taking place on Clapham Common on Midsummer Night's Eve 1991 at midnight. Clapham Common had been the scene of queer-bashing incidents, and OutRage! were invited to support the performance and sell whistles and organize a 'patrol' of the cruising ground.

More proactively, OutRage! decided to go to the centre of London's cruising life and set up a stall on Hampstead Heath in North London. The impetus came not only as an idea for outreach about the group, but also to offer some safer sex resources and, more cynically, as a fundraising event. On 16 August, the QUID subgroup set up its showcase stall late at night on the Heath, after agreeing to find a spot which wouldn't 'disturb' or intrude on the cruisers there.

They were planning on selling alcohol and I immediately stuck my hand up and said, 'Well, what's the point of giving away condoms?' All the leaflets said don't mix alcohol and sex! I thought this was ridiculous. I think it was at the time when I thought, fuck this.

MEGAN RADCLIFFE

They were a political group. I mean, safer sex came into it broadly. It was just another excuse for members of OutRage! to go cruising on the Heath. There was a bonfire that went out of control, completely out of control, we had to stamp on it. I'm surprised they weren't prosecuted.

JAMES KIERNEY

The Heath stall was very successful, with many men chatting to stall volunteers, and many whistles sold. OutRage! followed it up with a couple more stalls, precursors to some of the safer sex outreach now undertaken by groups such as Gay Men Fighting AIDS. Subsequently, Queer Heritage was set up by OutRage! members with an interest in Hampstead, not just as a cruising ground but also because of the Bathing Ponds, where many men swam naked during the summer. OutRage! also began organizing regular condom clear-ups of the Heath, following complaints from police, passers-by and the Heath wardens. They also distributed leaflets and protested at the continuing harassment of gay men using the bathing ponds following an incident when a man was arrested for wearing a T-shirt judged to be 'obscene' by the police. Although not all pond users were enthusiastic about OutRage!'s presence, they did attempt to build more constructive dialogue with users' committees and took a more active interest in the local Hampstead politics.

Hampstead Heath wasn't the only place with problems in the later part of 1991. A popular cruising ground further south, in Epsom, was also being targeted by the police, who had sent a letter to motorists using the Stew Ponds on the edge of Epsom Common, claiming that the area was a haunt for homosexuals, and was being used by parents of young children. The letter encouraged anyone with information to contact the police. In addition, the police mounted an operation involving at least half a dozen officers, many undercover, and arrested 28 people with fines of up to £1000 – ten times the usual amount for first time offences. The local paper, the *Epsom and Ewell Herald*, published the names and addresses of those arrested and sent a reporter along on a police operation:

As the *Herald* man walked around the paths with police, men could be seen walking slowly round the same routes and it was easy to see how visitors to the area feel intimidated and uncomfortable. The surveillance job is uncomfortable for male and female officers. Some have to lie still for hours watching a particular spot. The ground is often damp and covered in horse manure and they can be plagued by insects.[3]

In August, OutRage! member Martin Harrington decided that the police operation was breaching guidelines agreed by the London Policing Initiative Group. He went to Epsom to inform cruisers that the police were carrying out a surveillance operation, and was shocked when, approaching a man dressed in overalls open to the waist and apparently with nothing on underneath, he was himself arrested with obstructing the police. OutRage! zapped the cruising ground *en masse* on 21 August. Disappointed at not finding any police surveillance, they continued their protest at the local police station. Their demands included that the surveillance operation and pending prosecutions be dropped, that the police stop using *agents provocateurs*, and that the police justify the expense incurred in the operation.

Police would hide under a makeshift bunker that they'd put leaves over. We went to the cruising ground in the day and demolished them. There were a lot of things about transport. Epsom was a bit far out. There were very few people had cars. Some people went on the train, but if it involved travel a lot of queens said 'Oh, I can't be bothered.'

JAMES KIERNEY

They were going to the perverse lengths of tracing the car owners through their number plates and writing letters to their houses, effectively outing them to their families. So Martin Harrington arranged a very high-profile 'spot the cop' operation, where we went down with placards and re-enacted a number of events. I remember Martin Girvin, whose father is some high-up police officer, giving a police officer a right old slanging match, a 'Do-you-know-who-I-am' sort of conversation. I think Martin Harrington went back, subsequent to the action, and upset the police by continuing to point them out.

STEVE MAYES

The police operation did stop, and OutRage! claimed a victory after humiliating the police endeavours. Martin Harrington was acquitted on a technicality.

No such thing as bad press?

With both Hampstead and Epsom, the press had taken an interest in gay men's cruising activities – Epsom had given the press an opportunity to report on the police campaign, while the London *Evening Standard* chose to sensationalize the threat of cruising on the Heath in an article on 12 September. More significantly, on 7 September, in an article titled 'Gay Abandon', the allegedly liberal *Guardian* continued an apparent tradition of publishing negative articles about homosexuals. It infuriated not only OutRage!, but also some of the original members who had since 'left' or been ousted, particularly Steve Stannard and Dave Bunnett. They quickly formed an organization called Socialist Lesbians And Gays (SLAGS), a name which they knew would be anathema to the more hard-line OutRage! activists.

One Saturday afternoon, reading this awful article in the *Guardian*, myself and David Bunnett decided this was outrageous and we needed to do something about it, so we went and bought some software and produced a few leaflets.

STEVE STANNARD

We organized a picket outside the *Guardian*. It was that easy. We wouldn't have got the same response if there hadn't been OutRage! We didn't expect many people to turn up, although Derek Jarman did.

DAVE BUNNETT

OutRage! were very undecided until the night before the action. That was a turning point for the *Guardian*. They were shocked by the response. They got more critical letters around that article than any other single issue in the previous five years. They'd never been picketed about anything.

STEVE STANNARD

We demanded a meeting with Peter Preston, the editor, and we got it. We saw him briefly and a week later we spent two hours there. He took that issue seriously, and that did make an effect, slowly. He said he wasn't going to start recruiting gay journalists. OutRage! did a lot to raise those issues because there was a flurry of gay stuff in the media. None of that could have happened in a way without AIDS, because AIDS allowed people to start talking about gay sex, and everybody now knows what we do in bed, so we can have a Kiss-In and it's not an issue.

DAVE BUNNETT

Although OutRage! attended the picket of the *Guardian* offices in Farringdon Road, it also attempted a 'boycott' of the *Guardian* which was less successful. The picket was successful at embarrassing the paper, and ultimately in helping changing the nature of future reporting on homosexuality.

The general tone of media interest was beginning to shift, partly because of the high profile of spokespeople from groups such as Stonewall and OutRage! In August, OutRage! produced its own in-house paper, aimed at supporters and members, called *Queer Reality*, which carried articles on most of the major campaigns and focus groups. The paper was enthusiastically received at first, but was produced by a small group of people, notably Martin Harrington and Aamir Ahmed, and although there was a second issue, it never really took off in the way that was hoped.

It came about because there was and is a recognized need to communicate to members about what's happening and also outside the group to explain and tell people what's going on. It was also an attempt to try and harness some of the very disparate things that were going on all over the place. There was a list of affinity groups and a list of actions and objectives. It worked very well for one issue, unfortunately it was out of date by the time it was published. There was a limit to how much Martin and Aamir could do, and they were doing so many other things it was the first one to go, and no one else got involved.

STEVE MAYES

In the meantime, OutRage! was still struggling with internal tensions over its direction and style, and the growth of focus or special interest groups initiated a series of conflicts between policies and individuals which would only really be resolved over a year later.

NOTES

1 George Carey's first photo call on 27 July 1990, at the announcement of his appointment. Reported in the *Independent*, 28 July 1990.
2 That 'OutRage! were informed' about this is perhaps to disown my own involvement in the whole St Michael's affair. The Sisters of Perpetual Indulgence were approached by a TV documentary programme who wanted to expose the ex-gay movement through a video diary. They wanted to set up an action that they could follow with their cameras, in order to research the Living Waters ministry. At least, that's what they originally said. In fact, they felt it was too 'controversial' and although they fed a lot of information to us and OutRage!, they were scared that having one of the Sisters front their programme might be too 'biased', and opted instead to approach the Lesbian and Gay Christian Movement and some ex-gay people.
3 Quoted in *Capital Gay*, 'Activist arrested for warning innocent men', 23 August 1991.

SIX

Sequins, Labia, Children

With the success of affinity groups such as the Whores of Babylon, and the increasing influence from Queer Nation in America, the original OutRage! structure began to change significantly. Early on, an anti-censorship group, PUSSY (Perverts Undermining State ScrutinY), was founded, with its stated purposes being;

1. to fight sexism AND to promote sex – especially lesbian and gay sexualities

2. to fight the censorship of lesbian and gay sexual images – both by the state and within our own communities

3. to use direct action strategies – and to have a fabulous time – in the pursuit of these goals

4. to bring together people of all gender persuasions in this fight.[1]

PUSSY became involved in a number of *causes célèbres*, notably the debate within the lesbian community over photographer Della Grace's (now Del Grace) provocative collection of photographs, *Love Bites*, which many lesbian feminist bookshops had refused to stock. PUSSY made sure that this, and the radical pro-sex lesbian magazine *Quim*, were made available at their own stalls and pressured other bookshops such as Sisterwrite and Silver Moon to stock the publications.

I got a copy of *Love Bites*, and we decided that that was a good starting point for us. The thing that struck me about OutRage! with hindsight was that they were very much of 'somebody's done this. Let's react.'

Somebody's fucked up major big time, we will zap them! It never seemed to be 'Censorship is constant, we will go to Gay's the Word and ask them why they will stock gay male porn but they won't stock lesbian porn.' It was, 'We'll stand outside the shop.'

MEGAN RADCLIFFE

It was another fairly self-interested affinity group, pandering to a lot of different personal tastes and interests, fetishes even, of individual members, which was quite entertaining. It became quite factionalized because there were some strong-minded people trying to promote their own interests and it didn't have a particularly deep political analysis. Mandy Merck came along and talked to us, we had a number of seminars on the legal side, the moral side of censorship, but at the end of the day it seemed to boil down to just having fun, and what personal interests there were, rather than focused political activity. Della Grace, a tremendous self-publicist, and not a very strong photographer, has a real panache for getting herself noticed and getting herself seen. *Love Bites* was having problems at that time, and she quite shrewdly got a number of people on the bandwagon to bring publicity to all that. One of the things that I enjoyed about OutRage! was there were a lot of dyke initiatives and women's interests were particularly taken up there, which was a breath of fresh air.

STEVE MAYES

The emphasis on fun, and particularly queer pleasure, fitted in with the broader queer philosophy where old anxieties about gender roles were thrown out in favour of a more flexible sexual and social identity.

Work It Girl

The sense of fun with which PUSSY, mainly a lesbian-led anti-censorship affinity group, conducted its campaigns was echoed by the queenie part of OutRage! too. Following the example of urban glamour assaults in America, WIG (Work It Girl) attempted to claim queer space through 'urban drag' in mainstream venues. Their first launch against the sensibilities of the straight and narrow was attending the queer-friendly movie, *In Bed with Madonna*.

When they all went to watch the Madonna film, they all wore these labels saying things like 'fag' and 'dyke' and 'clit-licker' and it was like they were saying 'Fuck queer – now you've got to decide which one of these you want to identify as.' I loved walking down the street with those labels, and people looking – they couldn't say any of those things.

LYNNE SUTCLIFFE

Following the simple premise that queers are everywhere, WIG planned a shopping trip down Oxford Street to bedazzle fellow shoppers with queer fashion.

It was saying, 'Yes we're different – we may look the same as you, but we are very much different.' I thought 'Great, go for it!' Mark Silas was there in habit, being outrageous. It was all about visibility.

ALAN JARMAN

I had one of those very tight skirts that billowed at the bottom. Shane was in drag, Lofty was in drag, Patrick was in drag, Aamir was in drag. We went to Laura Ashley, we had a minute's silence for Laura because Laura Ashley had fallen down the stairs. We went and had a make-over in Selfridges, had tea in Fortnum & Mason's upstairs. That was queer visibility at its best.

JAMES KIERNEY

WIG was an action without any justification whatsoever. We tried very hard to make it into something legal, but failed abysmally. [It was] so empowering walking down Oxford Street and getting away with it. There was no attempt to explain to anyone what we were up to. It was just dykes leading each other around on chains and boys dressed as girls. I didn't drag up. I enjoyed everyone else dragging up but couldn't carry it off with any conviction whatsoever!

STEVE MAYES

My one initial thought was that the drag wasn't very good. The tourists were 'this is really cool' and I didn't see anybody with any bad reaction at all. I don't know if that was because it was on Oxford Street. I think that should have been regular. But again, it was Patrick and Lofty and they had to do all the work, and all they got was flak because they'd spelt something wrong on their flyer.

MEGAN RADCLIFFE

We set off quite happily to do all the shops but the police found out and we had to walk between two lines of police. They thought it was a major demonstration. They didn't like it at all. We ended up in one of the stores, and all the staff were gay so we were quite happy to be seen having a cup of coffee with all the police standing around wondering what on earth was happening. Everyone was rather surprised, but nobody was at the throwing us out stage.

BETH LANE

OutRage! wasn't just a campaigning group, but a social movement as well. OutRage! became part of the scene itself, fashionable and chic, with its range of 'queer' merchandizing including whistles, T-shirts, IDs and badges. They encouraged identification with them and as part of a Queer Nation. On 26 August, they achieved the dizzy heights of winning the annual Vauxhall Tavern Sports Day, against teams from other gay pubs and organizations. The trophy became another site for debates about the use of the word 'queer', with OutRage! threatening to change the title on the trophy to 'Queer Sports Day'.

I was the captain of the team. I did the Yard of Ale, and I drank all of that and threw up over the first row of people. We won the shield and someone in the office sat on it. We had to hand the shield back, but all the little things around it, saying who'd won, fell off it. I had to buy a replica shield and have the Vauxhall Tavern put on it, all the things on it, but because these little things around the side, Black Cap – 91, fell off, we didn't know who it was [who'd won each year]. We just made them up, so the shield they've got at the moment in the pub is not the true shield!

JAMES KIERNEY

Following the idea of claiming queer space, another OutRage! sub-group, Queers Asserting the Right to Ride Every Line Safely (QUARRELS), took up the issue of safety for lesbians and gay men on London's Underground transport system.

I remember working with Megan and Catherine. We had a tape that said Queer Safe Space and we roped whole sections of the carriages, which was fab, it was extraordinary. People just got on and they could only go in half the carriage because the other half was this queer space, with this collection of nuns. Donna came on it in full leather chained to Julie. We altered the adverts, we'd stolen quite a lot of the adverts from round the tube and queerified them – 'Dateline' we'd made two women. Loads of stickers everywhere, 'Dyke sat here'. We had music, whistles, drums, finger cymbals, lots of singing, chanting. I had an Underground hat. I remember that we got a letter from the Underground saying that if we used their symbol we'd get taken to court, because we used an Underground symbol as part of the Q, and they were very upset about that.

LYNNE SUTCLIFFE

Pricking their conscience

More fundamental issues were also at stake in autumn 1991. For many years, the human rights organization Amnesty International had refused to take on cases of people imprisoned because of their sexuality. In 1975, Danish gay and lesbian groups first lobbied Amnesty International, and the Danish Section of Amnesty first introduced the question of whether homosexuals should be covered as prisoners of conscience at the International Council meeting. Four reports looking at the issue were commissioned as more and more international sections of Amnesty favoured adopting homosexuals as prisoners of conscience, including Austria, Canada, Denmark, France, Greece, Netherlands, Sweden, the United Kingdom, and the United States.

The issue came to a head as the Amnesty International Council prepared to meet in Yokohama, Japan. In August 1991, a Turkish transvestite, Demet, was arrested in Istanbul, beaten and raped by a number of policemen, and imprisoned. Formerly a journalist, Demet had been at the forefront of a campaign against police brutality by Turkish transvestites. Pressure built for Amnesty to adopt Demet as a prisoner of conscience. The International Lesbian and Gay Association was already pressuring Amnesty, and a new OutRage! affinity group, Queer Planet, arose to develop an action against the London headquarters of AI on 30 August.

We turned up and with due theatricality chained Chris Woods and Lynne to the doors of Amnesty, sealed them shut, having very thoughtfully checked the fire exits in the event of anything going wrong, which impressed me also. It was very nicely thought through. We effectively sealed the building off. During the course of the action, it began to bite. The management of Amnesty sealed the building, refused to have any conversation. They effectively thought, keep your heads down, they'll just go away. We carried on shrieking and screaming, the police turned up, there was nothing they could do. People within the building got messages out. It reverted to stupid things like throwing bits of paper to give messages of support. They were doing this in fear, because they were forbidden by their managers to get in touch with us. Of course, that was fuel to the fire, because they were telling us 'We've been told not to talk to you.' So that got us really excited.

STEVE MAYES

There were so many easy points to make with Amnesty – 'What the fuck are you doing? You're supposed to be about human rights. It's about time you started campaigning for us as well.' It seemed then that things were so much rawer, things hadn't been said before. It was quite strange, it was this big, big liberal institution, and here we were, being really cold-shouldered and told to fuck off by them.

ROB KEMP

The drama of it was such that not only did we feel better because we'd made our point, it was very soundly argued with our megaphones, the arguments came in a continual stream. You could see people lighting up in the building, saying 'Yes, we recognize what you're saying.'

STEVE MAYES

Queer Planet originally had some connection with computers, that we could link up to other places in the world and wouldn't it be brilliant if we could all share our experience. Looking back on it, I'm curious as to why we ended up outside Amnesty. There only seemed to be three people who had access to that kind of computer which made it a bit of a club. It should have been shared and it wasn't. It was a mistake.

MEGAN RADCLIFFE

Get the Queen!

As the State Opening of Parliament approached in October, rumours began to fly around OutRage! that an affinity group was going to be set up to disrupt a major sporting spectacle to get attention for lesbian and gay civil rights. Much of the planning was taking place outside the Thursday general meetings.

I assume it was one of Peter's ideas, although I still don't really know. Harrington plucked at my sleeve at the end of the meeting and said 'Are you prepared to something really noble for the cause? Can't tell you what it is, might involve getting arrested.' At that stage, I was a decent liberal, before having become corrupted by OutRage! [I] saw myself as a letter writer, and an upstanding member of society. The thought of being arrested was deeply shocking, so I was slightly taken aback by this, but at the same time highly flattered. I was saying 'No no, you can't possibly do that,' and Martin was saying 'If Peter thought we ought to go to prison, then I think we ought to.' It took me a day to get over the shock at the prospect of getting arrested, realizing no one else was going to volunteer for this. Having thought about it rationally, it has to be done because it's not about waving placards in front of the queen, it's actually about civil liberties, the right to protest, the right to have your voice heard, all the civil rights wrapped around homophobia.

STEVE MAYES

Meetings were arranged secretly, with plans of central London pored over, escape routes planned out, strategies debated and sorted for the State Opening of Parliament on 31 October.

There was going to be a diversionary group at St Stephen's Gate, and while that diversionary group was making trouble down that end, the action group would somehow arrange for a ladder to climb the statue of Winston Churchill, drape a pink feather boa over him and hang placards. We managed to sort it out with a friendly photographer that his ladder would be next to the statue.

STEVE MAYES

We met outside Brief Encounter and Peter turned up in a little cap, as if it was a disguise. He was not going to walk with us. So, this little bunch of queers with these banners and stuff rolled up under their arms would not be, in any way whatsoever, connected with this man in a cap. But all the way from Brief Encounter to Parliament, he kept running up to us and saying 'Don't forget this, don't forget that.' He was like this big mother hen.

MEGAN RADCLIFFE

Peter was in disguise with a beret and spectacles and a false moustache. I couldn't believe it. We'd all come with our large tourist maps so we didn't look like Londoners. He led me through the streets of London desperately trying to be a tourist, walking nonchalantly at 100 miles an hour. It was like a cartoon, pointing in a feverish way at objects, anything, and his moustache, which fell off.

STEVE MAYES

There was some fuck-up. We thought the police knew who we were and why we were there. We mistimed it slightly, we didn't get the Queen. She was coming down as we had the banner up and the police just leapt on us. They frog-marched us off and we were basically told if we hung around we'd get arrested. I said I had to be back at work and I went!

MEGAN RADCLIFFE

The plan went wrong when we saw the ladder next to the statue. It wasn't a step-ladder at all, it was like a set of library steps. The signals all went wrong because the decoy group never turned up. Peter started giving covert signals like 'We're off, we're going to do it,' so we lunged for the statue, to those two steps, as if to climb the statue, utterly ridiculous. Fortunately we were arrested before we could make too much of an exhibition of ourselves. Honour was satisfied. We had a pre-prepared slogan that Peter had prepared, running along the lines of 'Legislate equality for all lesbians and gays now!', impossible to chant in an organized way as you were dragged off by the police. One of my peers in the media afterwards said it was the worst arrest he'd ever seen.

We were put in adjacent cells, and Peter immediately began to say 'I want to be in the same cell as my colleague.' The police kept us separate apparently for sexual reasons – they wouldn't put men and women in the same cell, but they were really confused by two queers. So while we were waiting, Peter was sitting in his cell with a bit of paper and a pencil, which you're allowed, drafting a bill to put before Parliament. I had my camera, which you're allowed to keep, taking pictures. Eventually they put us together, at which point my camera batteries ran out, so I couldn't get any pictures of Peter in the cell.

STEVE MAYES

A new PC format

The changes in structure which had started at the beginning of the year became more structurally formidable as the year ended. The overriding criticism of OutRage! as white, male and middle class, caused strong tensions within the group. More crucially, OutRage! attempted to incorporate a 'politically correct' recruiting policy for new, 'representative' members.

Despite having many women involved in the early days of OutRage!, the group was not seen to be taking women's issues seriously. Meetings were planned to look exclusively at the role of women and women's campaigns within OutRage! and there was an attempt to address women's issues within a main meeting. An earlier group within OutRage!, the Ladies' Excuse Me, had been initiated to develop campaigns for women, but failed to make any ground, largely because of lack of numbers.

By August, pressure was on to launch groups targeting particular interests. The 'focus groups' launched on 22 August became known as LINK associated with disability, the Working Class Group which didn't use an acronym, ETHNIC (Expanding The Non-Indigenous Contingent) involving non-white OutRage! members, and LABIA (Lesbians Answer Back In Anger) concerned with women's issues.

Looking back on it, I think it was a bit of a PC knee-jerk. OutRage! had constantly said we are a group for everybody. It felt like they felt they had to give this impression to the outside world that they were a totally undivided group – no matter who came along, they were part of OutRage! The general criticism of OutRage! and my criticism still was that it gives people these ideas but the reality is it's a white, middle-class, male group, always has been and always will be. We didn't feel there was any real positive energy behind us. It seemed like 'Oh, you want your own group, then have your own group, just don't bother us.'

MEGAN RADCLIFFE

I know what I feel, what I felt about family or community, and I couldn't get my message across at all. Everything was very politically correct. People weren't aware of the issues, had never come across them before.

AJAY

The Working Class Caucus was run by Ajay, who everyone had problems with, because he took the moral high ground on issues to do with gender and race. I remember we asked him what was 'working class' and he said 'I'm not going to get into a discussion about that now, but people who are, know.'

GRAHAM KNIGHT

I think I started to facilitate meetings somewhere round this point and I had a loud voice which was good, but sometimes people would say to people to speak up, and I remember Ajay saying that was a really classist thing to say, because some people hadn't been brought up in a class where they'd been brought up to speak loudly. That left me in a real quandary – to speak loudly or not. Talking to Ajay about it later and saying for me it's not a class thing, it's part of my job, I was taught to speak loudly because it's my job, I work with a theatre company.

LYNNE SUTCLIFFE

The disability group was a disaster, and produced a leaflet. We took Tim's guidance for the wording, which got us into trouble because it used the word 'handicapped'. We didn't know any of the issues at all.

GRAHAM KNIGHT

You'd have a report-back from the People of Colour group and Aamir would say 'Well, I had a meeting with myself and decided…' I don't think anyone was racist – anyone who was overtly racist would have been kicked out. They always, always went on that we were white middle-class males. We were, and that's where the birth of the 'Right Off Caucus' was born. The Right Off Caucus was basically any of the males that fitted into that group. Even Aamir was a member of the Right Off Caucus. It was an informal thing. It's probably where Queers Bash Back came from. There was a joke – everyone had to go through the facilitator, but the Right Off Caucus never went via the facilitator because they weren't a focus group!

JAMES KIERNEY

It was very easy sometimes to think 'Oh, we'd better do something on lesbian issues' whereas it was much more organic in LABIA because it was women discussing lesbian issues rather than the men. Some of the men were fascinated by the name because I think they thought 'Why are they angry?' Somebody said 'Well, I've never seen a woman naked, I don't know what a woman's bits look like, I don't know what a labia is!'

LYNNE SUTCLIFFE

The judge and the dildo

LABIA was the most successful of the focus groups, both in attracting numbers and in creating actions. On 21 September, Jennifer Saunders was imprisoned on two counts of indecent assault, burglary, handling stolen goods, assault and taking vehicles. The charges of indecent assault were brought by the uncle and father of a young woman, Rebecca Andrews, whom Saunders was alleged to have had a relationship with. The prosecution alleged that Saunders had seduced her by pretending to be a boy, 'Jimmy', concealing her gender by pretending to have a boil on one side of her chest and a cancer on the other, and using a dildo to make love with. The prosecution also alleged that oral sex had taken place. In summing up at the trial, Judge Jonathan Crabtree had said 'I suppose the two women would rather have been raped by some young man...' The remarks were enough to make the case a *cause célèbre* for lesbians, and LABIA began to organize around the case.

A complicating factor in LABIA's response to the Saunders trial was the unhappiness of the defendant and her counsel at having high-profile demonstrations which might prejudice the court against them. LABIA attempted to maintain support for Jennifer Saunders through attendance at court and letter writing, publicity and campaigning, but stopping short of major demonstrations. It was only after Judge Crabtree's comments that LABIA's anger could be unleashed, with an action at the Lord Chancellor's Department on 7 November.

We thought it was unfair to be in jail for something consensual that was obviously trumped up by her uncle. It made my skin crawl how somebody can stand in a courtroom and say 'She'd prefer to have been raped, surely.' As someone who's been raped, that's the most awful thing. We made a bit of a booboo because we turned up at the wrong place. We arranged to meet outside the Lord Chancellor's Office, but went to his Department's office and stood out there for five hours. That was cold! The reason that the blokes came along to Jennifer Saunders, and it was very sweet Martin and Aamir coming along, but it was like we needed a bit of protection. I was pleased with the way it went, we got loads of signatures, and we handed that in. We wanted to see the Lord Chancellor – he was two miles up the road! We got this stupid little letter back saying it was being considered. The next thing Justice for Women got involved and then she's released and LABIA had been forgotten.

MEGAN RADCLIFFE

Nine months after her sentence, in June 1992 Saunders won a High Court Appeal which reduced her six-year prison sentence to two years' probation. Speaking after the appeal, as she was safely ensconced in a nearby pub, Jennifer revealed the truth about the infamous 'strap-on dildo'. 'There never was no dildo. They thought there had to be a penis involved, so they said that about the dildo… My tongue was good enough.'[2]

Jennifer Saunders was a case that we got behind and I was quite glad that Cherry Smyth said that if we hadn't been around, nobody would have known about it. That's one of the best slaps on the back that I ever got. I wrote to Jennifer Saunders, sent her some clippings and told her what was going on, she wrote back to me. She's out now, and that's fine.

MEGAN RADCLIFFE

We've come for your children!

Ever since Section 28 and the spectre of the 'loony left', the issue of education and homosexuality had been a contentious issue exploited by media, politicians and religious zealots. For many OutRage! members, there was also a dichotomy between being involved in a gay activist group and working within an education setting; most often, even 'out' members of OutRage! were closeted while teaching or in classroom settings. Eventually, John Jackson, Peter Tatchell and a few other members of OutRage! began to form an affinity group, organizing under the title Sex Information for Schools, Students and Youth (SISSY).

SISSY began to look at distributing positive images around lesbian and gay sexuality within schools, acknowledging that very few young lesbians and gay men see positive images of themselves at school or in the media. Additionally, they wanted to make the information useful not only to lesbians and gay men but also to their heterosexual school friends.

It wasn't 'Are you gay?' It was 'Do you have a friend who thinks they might be?' They used Martin and Aamir and me and Catherine and they were quite friendly photos, quite cuddly *Hello*-type photos. I remember thinking if I was at school, I wouldn't have taken them if they said 'you...', I would have taken them if they'd said 'your friend...', that was a really good way to do it.

LYNNE SUTCLIFFE

Pro-gay leaflets were to be distributed outside school gates. In the first instance, OutRage! chose a school in North London, Haverstock Hill, which had a fairly liberal teaching policy. The first SISSY action took place on 27 November at lunchtime, just as children were leaving for their break.

I got completely out of my depth, simply because of the fact that I didn't have any idea it was going to snowball. I put my work number on the press release and I was getting a whole day of non-stop phone calls. I got into trouble for that. It was so embarrassing, they said 'Don't put the number on a press release again!'... We met at the tube station and went round the corner and there was this total media scrum. We had to ask the police to move them back. They were round the entrance to the school; television cameras, flash photographers everywhere, reporters, microphones. It was a great success – it raised a lot of important issues that hadn't been talked about previously, they tried to brush it under the carpet. After that action, the school approached us and said, 'Have you got any young lesbian or gay people you can send in for a talk?', which we did and there were some really good responses. I wish somebody had done it for me.

JOHN JACKSON[3]

I started thinking about what it meant to the kids I was teaching at school and I thought if I was going around to schools, I had to be out in my own school. My 15-year-old boys were a bit giggly, but they saw a programme I was in.

LYNNE SUTCLIFFE

The action at Haverstock Hill caused immense controversy within the press, and OutRage! was criticized by every gay group, especially Stonewall. Undeterred, OutRage! continued the Schools actions, although they dropped the name SISSY and started up a YOUTH group. The OutRage! office received a significant number of enquiries from schoolchildren, and some new members to OutRage! came out as a result of having heard about the group through the controversial actions.

Early in the New Year, on 22 January 1992, OutRage! planned a similar action at Sacred Heart School in Camberwell in response to the 1991 draft *Catechism for Adults* which condemned lesbian and gay relationships. OutRage's! decision to leaflet the school brought a sharp press release from the Catholic Media Office, keen to point to statements from the Catholic Church condemning violence or discrimination against homosexuals:

The Church has a serious responsibility to work towards the elimination of any injustices perpetrated on homosexuals by society. As a group that has suffered more than its share of oppression and contempt, the homosexual community has a particular claim upon the concern of the Church.[4]

OutRage! was attempting to show how lesbian and gay students needed support against victimization in school, referring to a 1984 survey of 416 lesbian and gay teenagers by the London Gay Teenage Group that one in five of those questioned had attempted suicide. The idea to leaflet the school came from an unexpected source:

There was a teacher who was gay who suggested we do that school. He got pretty much hounded out after that.

JOHN JACKSON

Camberwell has a very high black population, and a lot of these kids were black – that, for me, was an issue, because of my visibility as a black person. I felt ridiculed by these children, because they didn't understand me at all. If anybody apart from a white man is gay, then it's the white man that's made them gay.

ALAN JARMAN

A lot of children did take leaflets, and a lot were supportive. A lot were giggling, but they were probably most interested and too embarrassed to let their friends know. We collected up the younger members of OutRage!, teenagers if possible, who'd just left school, to stand at the gates, and the rest of us would stand a bit further away, not to be too intimidating. Alan Jarman was standing next to Danny, handing out leaflets.

NICK CAVE

There was a woman who came up to us and threw this purple liquid in my face. I was completely horrified, thinking 'Shit! Somebody's killed me with acid' and it turned out to be vinegar. That was a bad experience for me. Because of that action, it brought a reaction. It wasn't something people appreciated – I felt I'd achieved something by provoking that reaction. That was probably one of the most frightening things I'd ever done.

ALAN JARMAN

We gave a lot of information out to schoolchildren. I remember covering the phones in the office, we were getting other schools from up north phoning us up, asking for copies of the leaflet, so they could copy it and give it to their schoolchildren.

NICK CAVE

For OutRage!, it had been a good year: a higher profile, more 'diversity' within the group, and a significant programme of events and campaigns for the first half of 1992, centring upon the country's upcoming general election. That campaign would prove to be another significant chapter in OutRage!'s history – 'Equality Now!'

NOTES

1 Handout 'ANNOUNCING A NEW OUTRAGE! AFFINITY GROUP...', launch of PUSSY, 23 May 1991.
2 'Judge frees jailed lesbian', Cherry Smyth in *Capital Gay*, 19 June 1992.
3 I was involved in the Haverstock Hill zap, and remember Peter Tatchell begging me not to let the Sisters attend in their habits. The day of the zap, a fundamentalist Christian stood over the road from us with a placard denouncing us and scared the kids. Many of the kids stopped and talked, particularly about how sad they felt for teachers they knew who were gay but couldn't come out. Some of them even took our OutRage! badges to wear. A week or so later, I was travelling on the tube and was approached by a girl who recognized me from the demo. She said how much she'd appreciated it and I met her on a later occasion, when she told me that one of her friends had come out to her after the demonstration, and she was glad we'd helped her to be open and supportive of her friend. See, every little bit helps...
4 1979 English and Welsh Bishops' pastoral guidelines, section 13, quoted on Catholic Media press release, 'Catholic Church Counters OutRage! Attack', 21 January 1992.

SEVEN

Equality Now!

In October 1991, Peter Tatchell proposed that OutRage! should conduct an extensive campaign around law reform and lesbian and gay equality which would culminate in a mass demonstration at the time of the General Election. The original proposal clearly aligned the new campaign – a move away from individual 'zaps' to a coordinated and lengthy campaign – with the struggles of other civil rights movements, such as the suffragettes, involving non-violent direct action and civil disobedience. Further,

> It ought to seek to undermine the moral legitimacy of homophobic oppression by forcing the State authorities to repress our just campaign for equality; thereby exposing the homophobic nature of the State and helping to evoke public sympathy for our cause.[1]

Equality Now was demanding proactive assertion of the civil rights of lesbians and gay men. The early ideas were radical and confrontational:

- ▲ A 24-hour 'Hunger-Strike For Lesbian & Gay Equality' outside Downing Street in mid-January; possibly followed by a longer hunger-strike a couple of months later.

- ▲ 'Kiss-In' style events to challenge specific homophobic laws, such [as] a 'Procuring Party', 'Cruise-In', 'Buggery Ball', and 'Right To Love' protest.

- ▲ Occupations and disruptions of big political, sporting and cultural events.

▲ A march on Parliament (in defiance of the Sessional Orders) at lunchtime on the first Monday of every month, beginning on 3rd February, to demand equal rights.[2]

The slogans prepared included 'Lesbian & Gay Equality Now', 'Free Lesbian & Gay Political Prisoners', and 'Repeal All Anti-Gay/Anti-Lesbian Laws'. Debates about the programme highlighted its emphasis on male issues and the amount of time and commitment such a campaign would need, at the expense of other actions. There were doubts within the group as to whether OutRage! could manage the campaign and whether this was the most useful way to devote its time and energy. There was also concern about some of the actions, such as going on hunger strike, or breaking the law in order to get arrested, particularly as the final point in the Equality Now proposal stated:

We should aim to encourage as many of those arrested as possible to refuse to pay fines and to go to prison. This will not be a stand that many people will feel able to take (because of job commitments and other reasons). However, even if only a few people were prepared to refuse to pay fines, it would still be of great symbolic value. The idea behind refusing to pay fines is to reject compliance with a homophobic State and refuse to accept that such a State has any right of authority over us while it continues to enforce laws which violate lesbian and gay human rights.[3]

Equality Now was just the dreariest campaign. It turned OutRage! into a sub-suffragette organization. It stripped out its soul. It committed it to a rolling programme of action upon action that took away its creativity and its independence of thought and its radicalism.

CHRIS WOODS

I felt that it was a real turning point for OutRage!, because it turned away from any attempt at participatory community politics into a purely media event. It happened at difficult times of the week, like one o'clock on a Thursday when most people couldn't make it.

GRAHAM KNIGHT

I went through it at the meeting and I just felt, for an equality thing, do you want gay male equality with straights? Lesbians with gay men? It felt like a personal vision. There was a lot in the Equality Now thing that I didn't agree with, and I put my hand up and said so. I got shot down quite a lot. I think people realized I was a bit of a mouth.

MEGAN RADCLIFFE

This was where Peter really proved himself to me, in that the philosophy behind it was so sound, although some of the actions themselves were either silly or weren't organized as well as they could have been. The philosophy behind it, of being proactive, of actually raising issues around sexuality before they were on the media's agenda, [it was] the first time I was aware of this being done.

STEVE MAYES

At the time I arrived, Equality Now was the main business of the group and I had no reason to believe it was being contested, or had been contested. I came in a hand-over period. There seemed to be a new dominant group appearing in Equality Now.

STEVE COOK

The Equality Now campaign was adopted, although Peter's original proposals were altered and the timetables rearranged. Tuesday evenings became a time for a 'steering' or organizing group to meet. Very quickly, the Tuesday Group attracted all those who were interested in the campaign and, because of the nature of the campaign, became a tightly knit group itself.

The Tuesday meeting was anybody who wanted to help. Because people were together regularly for a long series of months, we came out a fairly well lubricated machine, and as the rest of OutRage! petered away, you were left with this machine in working order, while other things fell off.

FERNANDO GUASCH

Arrest me, arrest me!

The opening demonstration for Equality Now was planned to be a show of civil disobedience, claiming both a right to a democratic voice and to equal rights for lesbians and gay men. A March on Parliament to Reclaim Lesbian and Gay Human Rights was called for 6 February 1992, starting at Bow Street Police Station. The nature of the demonstration – a mass protest outside Parliament while Parliament sits – could be interpreted by the Police as an illegal act, breaking the 'Sessional Orders'. In order to minimize problems with the police, OutRage! began a campaign to inform the police of all their actions. The first contact was Peter, a role later taken up by Nick Cave:

I'd usually have a chat with Peter before I'd go along to meet the police at Cannon Row, Chief Inspector Ashwell. We wouldn't always tell the police the whole story. I'd have to fill out a form, to give notice that we intended to do a demo, give the police an idea of what's required, give them the route of the march. They would take that away, say thank you very much. A fortnight later, they'd ask me to pop in, say you can't stop at that place there. Usually I'd agree to it, although if it was something we really, really wanted, I'd say 'We'll cut it short if you allow us to do this one thing.' It was a bit of a game, really. We'd demand more than we actually wanted, at the next meeting we'd discuss it and come to an agreement. The police said, 'If you pass this point here, we'll arrest you' and I turned round and said 'You'll find if you arrest us here, further down the street, you'll keep the traffic flowing. It's better for us for our pictures and it's better for you to keep the traffic flowing.' They actually took advice from us on some occasions.

NICK CAVE

Given that the size of 'OutRage!' demonstrations was usually very small by comparison with other protests that the Metropolitan Police routinely dealt with, the initial meeting consisted of a large number of officers and the rank of its chairman (a Commander) testified to the seriousness with which the group was viewed – 'OutRage ' were trouble. The organiser – an articulate man, active in left-wing Labour Party politics – was precisely the type of person with whom the police least preferred to negotiate... He pointed out that [the Sessional Order] prohibited *disorderly* gatherings and *obstruction* of free access to the Palace of Westminster, and that the proposed protest would satisfy neither criterion. However, [the police] insisted that, given the record of 'OutRage!' demonstrations, police were entitled to apprehend that the march might be disorderly and therefore it would not be permitted within the Sessional Area.[4]

The aim of the march was to secure as much media attention as possible, and OutRage! knew that peaceful protestors being arrested would make headlines. In addition, the involvement of celebrities such as Derek Jarman and Jimmy Somerville would attract the press. At all stages of the protest, it was made very clear that as soon as the march turned into Leicester Square, those taking part would be breaking the law and would be arrested by the police, but probably (OutRage! hoped) released without trial. A leaflet giving legal guidelines was given out, including advice on arrest, by a gay-friendly solicitor/OutRage! member. Further advice included:

While you are being processed by the Custody Sergeant, you should point out that our protest action was completely peaceful, caused no damage, involved no offensive language or behaviour, was good natured and courteous, and concerned the exercise of our legitimate right to demonstrate.[5]

The march assembled at Bow Street Police Station where Labour MP Jeremy Corbyn called for legislation to end discrimination on the grounds of sexual orientation. The march continued towards Parliament. There was a brief pause as an arrest was made, a busker at Leicester Square tube station unconnected with OutRage! A pink ribbon, marking the boundary of the 'Sessional Area', was cut ceremonially by Stephen Lind dressed as Margaret Thatcher. The police and OutRage! stewards warned people that if they progressed further, they would be arrested.

There were a number of celebrities on the march and they were at the front holding a large banner. The police commander instructed TSG [Territorial Support Group] officers to make arrests from the rear of the sit-down towards the front row so as to allow the celebrities maximum exposure to the news media. TSG officers went to each protestor in turn and, in a carefully rehearsed operation, repeated the warning, asked if the person understood the warning, asked them to move and when they refused arrested them All of this was filmed by a police video crew.[6]

People were told if they didn't want to get arrested, they should step out, and that left 60–70 people who went off to Charing Cross Road. Everybody lay down, arms locked, and waited to be arrested, in an orderly way. There were loads of cameras, the police gave time for the media to take pictures. I was put in a van, taken down the police station, processed and cautioned. It was my first arrest and I think through sheer middle-class arrogance, I didn't have a problem with it, because we pay police people's wages! I'd also taken the day off work.

STEVE COOK

My most enduring memory of that day is of being arrested and carted off in this police van. I was at Kennington Police Station and I was the first person taken in. I ended up sharing the cell with three other gay men, which was amazing, and one of them was Terry Sanderson,[7] and we just sat and gossiped all the time. I was the first one out as well, and I spent most of the time in the cell writing a press release.

JOHN JACKSON

I was alone in a cell for an hour and a half. They let me out, told us we were going to be given a caution. It was only after going to the Thursday meeting we realized by accepting a caution we were pleading guilty. They didn't charge us with breaking the Sessional Orders, they just charged us with obstruction. The only one who didn't accept a caution was Martin Girvin, whose dad was the Chief Constable of Wiltshire.

JOHN BEESON

The question now arose about what further action should be taken. Initially, it had been thought likely that all those arrested would be charged. However, the cooperation shown by the organizer was now thought to justify less severe action and all those arrested were released without charge. Police were gratified to receive the thanks of the organiser, some celebrities, and other protestors for their handling of the event. This gratitude was repeated in a magazine article by one of the celebrities that police displayed with a mixture of incredulity and pride when I next visited the Special Events office.[8]

The first Equality Now action had been a tremendous success, gaining national coverage in all media with 45 people. There was international interest in the campaign, much of which covered in greater detail what the national press only touched upon – the civil rights of lesbians and gay men in Britain.

Queer soldiers

The next Equality Now action was the most contentious within the group, arguing for equality for lesbians and gay men in the military. It was an action which many members felt they couldn't support for pacifist reasons, while others felt strongly for it, often because of personal experience.

I did a lot of the research work on it, liaising with Rank Outsiders and Stonewall. The reason for that was that my brother was a Staff Sergeant in the Royal Engineers and I had an interest in the army through that. I didn't want to serve in the armed forces. I'm quite happy if I'm barred. One of my closest friends was thrown out of the Air Force for being gay. He wanted to stay in that job, he didn't want to be thrown out, although after his interrogation he was happy to leave. He had sleep deprivation, was quite badly mistreated.

NICK CAVE

I was a nurse in the military for nearly seven years and I didn't come out in the military. I spent the last two years at the recruiting depot, where whoever came out was severely punished. I just kept myself under wraps, but I could see the damage done to everybody else. Girls were being thrown out left, right and centre, and I had to do their medicals. I thought I'd better keep quiet, because it'll be me next time.

BETH LANE

Robert Ely [of Rank Outsiders] at first wasn't that happy to be involved because he thought it might damage his organization, because they rely on complete confidentiality. They didn't really want their name to be associated with a big high-profile demo. They gave us a lot of help, they put us in touch with people who were prepared to be on the demo and to speak out on the demo.

NICK CAVE

The idea was to 'reclaim' or queerify military leaders who were thought to be gay or bisexual. OutRage! planned to approach statues of famous allegedly gay military leaders – Kitchener, Haig, Montgomery and Mountbatten – and to hand in a letter of protest to the Secretary of State for Defence, Tom King. The letter detailed the 'undesirable effects' the military ban on homosexual Service personnel had, including the encouragement of abuse and maltreatment, reinforcing social prejudice, contradicting the policies of other NATO countries and the discouragement of effective HIV prevention education. Press releases highlighted statistics showing that between 1987 and 1990, 306 lesbians and gay men were dismissed from the armed forces, and 32 were imprisoned for up to two years, even where consensual relations took place with civilians outside of barracks during off-duty hours. The statues were covered in pink feather boas, or had a speech bubble held next to them, saying 'Can Kill, Can't Love a Man'.

I nearly got arrested first off. They told me later, they didn't know whether I was a civilian or military, in my nursing uniform, and they didn't know whether to arrest me when I arrived. As I was actually speaking to the press, because I'd been in the military, they didn't know what to do about me.

BETH LANE

I was personally very unhappy about supporting the military. Equality Now was about publicizing an area of the culture that was homophobic. I never could understand the ratio of work to the amount of publicity you'd get. The military action was a really boring zap to us, but got amazing publicity.

DAVID ARNOLD

We finally laid a wreath at the Ministry of Defence. The basic idea I think is if you're queer you can serve during wartime because we need you, but we don't need you in peacetime, so you can sod off. They'll let us die for our country, but they won't let us serve our country in peacetime.

NICK CAVE

One of the longest, most boring, coldest demonstrations I have ever been on. We had to walk around all the statues of the people we were outing. There's a statue in Whitehall, Kitchener possibly, and David was the only one tall enough to hold this speech bubble on an extremely long pole to come out of his mouth. This historian, who'd written an autobiography I think of Mountbatten's wife, was on TV and said 'I'm always hearing stories... there's not a shred of evidence. He liked women. He had three daughters!' If Edwina Mountbatten wasn't aware that he was homosexual, the biographer wouldn't be either. English men have this homosexual thing, in that they like other male company, they don't like women, and particularly that Edwardian Empire thing. There was twitching of curtains at the Ministry of Defence, which they caught on film wonderfully.

MARTIN MAYNARD

Nudge, nudge, wink, wink

The success of the first two Equality Now actions had led to a very high media profile for OutRage!, and for queer issues. OutRage! were always conscious of their own successes, actions which had worked well in the past. The Kiss-In was still talked about enthusiastically, and it was the most obvious action to 're-visit' during Equality Now. As an extension of the theme, the action would focus on laws affecting cruising and procuring, emphasizing the effects of Section 32 of the 1956 Sexual Offences Act, originally introduced to combat heterosexual men seeking female prostitutes, but often used against gay men. In 1989, in England and Wales, 462 men were convicted and 117 cautioned for cruising and chatting up other men. Six of them were imprisoned and three received sentences of between 6 and 12 months.

The 'Wink-In' on 5 March 1992 aimed to provide a fun forum to flout the law, and demonstrate against arrests of gay men for cruising, chatting-up, winking, smiling and exchanging names and phone numbers. A collection of elaborate props were constructed by the OutRage! handymen, Martin Corbett and John Beeson, including large 'winking' eyes on sticks, large placards with telephone numbers on to exchange, and the erection of a Wendy house to contain and conceal 'bonk-ins' involving more than two gay men.

Looking back at it now, being arrested for giving someone your phone number seems a little bit ridiculous, but I can remember when people were done for it. Some of the phone numbers that were held up on big boards were government ministries, Downing Street and things like that.

It was terribly theatrical. We stood on the Eros statue and publicly kissed, winked and exchanged phone numbers.

MARTIN MAYNARD

I remember swapping a very large phone number with my name and the Conservative Party Headquarters number on, not my own.

FERNANDO GUASCH

We had to hold on to the rails on the inside of this Wendy house and just rock it from side to side, and drop our trousers, as if something was happening. The police were very interested. I remember this policeman looking underneath to see what was going on.

JOHN JACKSON

I doubt it had any effect at all on the laws, but in terms of making people aware how silly they were, I guess it had some kind of effect.

GRAHAM KNIGHT

It was inspired, such a stupid and banal idea, about a profoundly important subject. The statistics to back it up were shocking. The idea of taking a banal activity such as winking I thought was very shrewd.

STEVE MAYES

The whole enterprise was extremely light-hearted and, although the officer in charge kept a close eye on the proceedings to ensure that decency was maintained, no attempt was made to restrain the protest. On the contrary, the complaints of a few bystanders were ignored and building workers near the scene were instructed to stop taunting the protestors.[9]

The action finished with a lobby of Members of Parliament and was backed up with a letter delivered to all the political party leaders demanding to know if they would support a series of ten measures aimed at eliminating discrimination. The letter was signed by Derek Jarman, Tom Robinson and Jimmy Somerville. It finished:

We would appreciate receiving your detailed reply to each of these 10 legislative proposals so we can communicate your party's policies to the estimated 12.5 million lesbian, gay and bisexual citizens of this country – many of whom will shortly vote in the forthcoming general election.

Thank you. We take the courtesy of informing you that a copy of this letter is being released to the lesbian and gay press and to the national media – as will a copy of your reply.[10]

Married bliss?

The letter to the MPs had included a desire for legislative reform to give legal recognition and protection of same-sex relationships through a system of 'registered partnerships' which would grant registered lesbian and gay couples the same legal rights as married men and women. Whereas 1991's Queer Wedding had been a set-up, with partners who weren't even going out with each other, the Equality Now action took long-term relationships and made applications to register them at Westminster Registry office.

The right to marry and found a family is a fundamental human right. It's wrong to deny that right to the thousands of people who are in committed same-sex relationships. If Lynne gets sick, I'd want to be able to get compassionate leave from work to care for her. In the event of Lynne having an accident or dying, we both want the law to recognize her as next of kin. When I worked as a nurse, I saw the partners of lesbian and gay patients excluded from the hospital bedside by parents who disapproved of their relationship. There were instances where hospital staff ignored the wishes of homosexual patients and their partners. They took the side of homophobic parents who were granted next of kin status and abused that position to deny the wishes of their lesbian and gay children.

SARAH HEWS

We desperately had to chase round and find top hats and tails and things, and remember I'm 5' 7¾" and David is six foot! We had to have it guaranteed by a credit card as well, and I'd just lost mine. We rang round everyone, no one had a credit card, except Shaun Steppie eventually. On the morning we got all dressed up. Martin Corbett picked us up. As luck would have it, it was the day Fergie and Andy announced that they were going to get divorced, and that was the first of the royal divorces.

MARTIN MAYNARD

The registrar was in a complete panic. We'd done everything totally properly, we'd got our birth certificates, our £15 and we'd put our applications in the week before. They knew we were coming, but they didn't expect us in our dresses and with our flowers. I think I had a little fantasy as we went in that they were going to say yes, OK you can get married. We had two witnesses and her saying 'I'm really sorry, I can't marry you' and us saying 'Why, why can't you marry us?' She said 'It's against the law', and I said 'What law?' She got down the book and she was trying to find the exact statute. It was a very old dusty book, like a prop, turning the pages with dust flying off. I thought it was very symbolic that it was all dusty, and me going 'I'm so disappointed, are you sure you can't marry us?'

LYNNE SUTCLIFFE

It then broke up – people had forgotten to bring the champagne. We bought it for ourselves. We were on the dole, we had to buy our own champagne for our own mock wedding!

DAVID ARNOLD

Very shrewd, it didn't pander to the sentimental garbage about marriage. It was about legal recognition of partnerships for very pragmatic reasons – insurance, property, very rooted on real identifiable, quantifiable issues. The couples were serious about registering their partnerships and it was a very confrontational action. Along with the other OutRage! actions, it lives on now, through the photos which are still used on a regular basis and the fact that it's still talked about.

STEVE MAYES

We had to get up at some God-forsaken hour, five o'clock, get into our glad rags again [for a television debate]. I'd actually said to the guy, do you mind if I take my Bible in with me, because I know my Bible, and I knew somebody was going to bring it up. At one point, a black evangelical Christian woman cried out 'It says in the Bible man shall not lie with man! I managed to get the eye of the presenter and I had my Bible there and I had it marked and I went 'Yes, it also says…' I was desperately trying to find a ridiculous one, and managed to find 'They who trim their beards and cut their locks shall be accursed in the sight of the Lord. How many people here shaved this morning?' Someone said to me afterwards, if it came to choose your neighbours out of the two groups, they'd like the gay boys. Our downstairs neighbours, a very old lady, I bumped into her a couple of weeks later and [she] thought we were very good. Just after that I went to an off-licence to get some wine and the guy there said 'I saw you on TV. My neighbour did and he still wants to live next to you.'

MARTIN MAYNARD

Three in one

OutRage! achieved a remarkable feat for their next demonstration. Not content with one demonstration against employment discrimination, on 2 April three actions occurred centred on the same theme. Several prominent employment discrimination cases were being featured in the mainstream media, most notably the case of police officer Alison Halford, who had been denied promotion nine times and had been the subject of disciplinary proceedings. A number of anti-gay comments had been made about her by police officers and Liverpool councillors, and it was revealed that James Sharples, Merseyside's Chief Constable, had been keeping a file on Halford referring to her 'improper' relationship with another woman. OutRage! accused the police of homophobia, and organized an action outside Scotland Yard, preceded by a picket of the Department of Employment while wearing uniforms from different professions. The picket was addressed by Sarah Cunningham, an ex-Metropolitan Police officer who claimed to have been forced out of the police because of her lesbianism, Reverend Michael Peet, a gay priest, and the veteran lesbian rights and peace campaigner Pat Arrowsmith.

OutRage! handed in a letter to the Department of Employment which highlighted a Lesbian and Gay Employment Rights survey finding in 1986 that 25 per cent of lesbians and gays had experienced discrimination in their workplace, with 6 per cent having been dismissed from their jobs because of their sexual orientation. The letter went on to state:

Other European countries recognise homophobia in employment as a serious problem which merits legislative remedy. The Netherlands, France, Sweden, Denmark and Norway have extended their anti-discrimination protection to prohibit discrimination against lesbians and gay men – as befits democracies committed to upholding human rights and treating all citizens equally.

We urge you to follow their positive example by drawing up legislation to ban employment discrimination against lesbians and gay men; thereby giving us the same protection that successive governments have long given to women and black people.[11]

I had this idea from the suffragettes, to try and get people to parade with placards of their professions. 'Women can do scuba-diving, women can be doctors', dress up. It was one of our most boring actions. It was a picket.

FERNANDO GUASCH

Everyone was dressed up in different professions, there was this police woman who talked about being assaulted by the police. Ultimately, we discovered it was all not true.

DICE

The dullness of the pickets was contrasted sharply with another event which took place almost by accident. Australian ex-soap star and singer Jason Donovan was involved in a libel trial against fashion magazine *The Face*, which had reproduced the image of Donovan wearing a *Queer as Fuck* T-shirt. Knowing that Donovan was at court, some members of OutRage! hung around waiting to catch him.

I can remember hanging around for a long, long time. I remember Jason coming out of the court. I said to him, 'I hope you'll give support to the lesbian and gay community by accepting OutRage!'s offer to come on a benefit', and he said 'Yeah, I'll do that, mate.'

DICE

It was absolutely off the cuff, unthought out other than the fact that Peter realized Jason Donovan was going to be outside court with cameras, let's be there. That five minutes of standing with placards behind Jason's head had a real impact. I see those pictures being used again and again and again. People will always talk about that case, people are still doing that with the Liberace case against the *Daily Mirror* and that was years ago. People will be talking about the Jason Donovan case for years: every time they will use a picture taken outside court and there isn't a picture in existence without an OutRage! poster behind him, a queer-affirming OutRage! poster.

STEVE MAYES

Infiltrating Downing Street

Equality Now had been organized before the date of the General Election had been announced. After John Major was re-elected, some members of OutRage! decided to pay him a little visit to 'congratulate' him on his success. A small group of protesters arrived at Downing Street and joined a collection of people awaiting the newly elected Prime Minister.

We had posters up our sleeves; they searched us and they didn't search our sleeves, it was all really spooky. There was a whole bank of press in Downing Street and we were right at the front, near a barrier, and I thought we'd be able to get a brilliant photograph. The only people in front of us were people from Conservative Headquarters and lots of pretty blond girlies, going to me 'Isn't it exciting!' and me going 'It's so exciting!'

Tim, standing right beside me, they asked him to move. I said to them 'Why do you want him to move?' I knew why, because the Prime Minister is going to come out any second and he was going to come and shake hands with these pretty girls and they didn't want Tim in the photograph. They'd deliberately got all these beautiful people at the front, John Major's kind of Britain, and Tim didn't fit in. He got very upset, because he knew that he hadn't done anything wrong. The police were saying he's got to move and they started to move him physically and led him away. I started to say 'You can't take him out, he's done nothing wrong' and they started to say 'She's a troublemaker' and 'Hold the Prime Minister' because he was just about to come out. I said to Hannah, 'I'm going to get thrown out.' She said 'We may as well go for it now', so I took the poster out of my sleeve and held it up. People were ripping it down. Hannah and Tanya held theirs up, there was pandemonium, the press was going wild. I got dragged off by a load of policemen, elbowed in the nose, and they must have got some good shots that day, but not one of them was used at all. Nobody mentioned it.

LYNNE SUTCLIFFE

The action was reported by the gay press, but not by the mainstream. The protesters did get a round of applause at the next OutRage! meeting, however.

Bend over for your Member

The pressure behind the OutRage! campaign was intense, with a major action every fortnight. The effect was both tiring and demoralizing, as the press attention waned after the election had been won by the Conservatives. Many of the Equality Now actions were about providing photo opportunities to the press in order to raise and discuss issues around lesbian and gay civil rights. For the issue of the unequal age of consent, OutRage! chose to adopt a traditional Maori insult. The plan to 'Drop your trousers and bend over for your Member' involved a group of men exposing their boxer shorts, with 'Equality Now' spelt out, and then pointing their posteriors at Parliament. The plan was to then move the demonstration from Parliament to Cannon Row police station, where protestors would 'confess' to having under-age sex, and call for the police to arrest them. The event started with a letter being delivered to the Home Office at Queen Anne's Gate, which detailed OutRage!'s case for an equal age of consent.

I was the letter E I think. Part of it was a march to the Home Office, and we went there and stood outside and then went on to Parliament. Someone produced these boxer shorts which spelt out 'Equality Now'. We went to the toilets below Whitehall and changed into them. Someone changed in the middle of the toilet area, with nothing on. I was more modest and went into a cubicle.

DICE

I wasn't one of the bending over group, but I stood at the end with a placard. That picture was quite widely used, and it did annoy some Tory MPs. There were some quite militant young boys who'd come down from up North, and there was a snog outside one of the government departments.

GRAHAM KNIGHT

The police had warned us that everybody would get arrested if anybody showed their bare bums.

JOHN BEESON

When they dropped their trousers outside Parliament with the letters stuck to their bottoms, I thought they'd lost it. I didn't want to be part of it. It was cheap.

JAMES KIERNEY

Homo promo

The penultimate demonstration for Equality Now was an easy target. Section 28 of the Local Government Act had long been resented since its introduction in 1988, making it illegal for local governments to finance the 'promotion' of homosexuality. The law had not led to court action but there were several instances of self-censorship, where local councils had prevented homosexuality from being discussed or 'advertised'. The seventh Equality Now action aimed to directly challenge the thinking behind the law, by providing a 'free trial offer' of homosexuality. A later parade with posters including slogans such as 'Once ridden... Forever Smitten', 'Lesbian Sex... Finger Licking Good', 'Cock S**king... The Taste Of A New Generation', 'Gay Sex... It's the Real Thing' and 'Dyke... Just Do It' was organized outside Parliament. Gay 'beefcake' and lesbian 'cheesecake' were also free to offer themselves as Free Trial Samples. Although initially advertised to attend, the lead singer of pop group Right Said Fred, Richard Fairbrass, failed to attend.

It was me and Mark smooching outside Tory Party HQ, and I think Daniel Curry made a speech which took the piss out of Tory activists. It was basically a taunting.

STEVE COOK

He made a speech why queens were much better than heterosexuals, and Linda Bellos, who'd made a speech before Daniel's, freaked out. She said it was disgraceful, too strong.

FERNANDO GUASCH

Naughty, naughty, naughty

The relationship with the police throughout the Equality Now campaign had been very good. However, with the opening of a new Parliament, OutRage! came into direct conflict with them. The police expressly forbade OutRage! to have any sort of demonstration, and asked for any details of a demonstration in advance. On 6 May, the State Opening of Parliament, they came across a press release from OutRage! saying that the group planned to break the police ban. OutRage! had previously asked for a copy of the Commissioner's Directions for the event, which stated that anyone displaying banners or placards would be arrested immediately.

OutRage! argued that the ban was a fundamental denial of civil rights and the right to protest. The police were insistent that they would not let any demonstration take place, and that any demonstrators would be arrested. On the day, the police identified a small group of OutRage! protesters, and as they prepared to unfurl banners as the Queen approached, they were immediately leapt on by police officers. A second demonstration was dealt with similarly.

Whereas the police were prepared to be tolerant and accommodating towards what they regarded as bona fide protest demonstrations, the threat of in-the-job trouble resulting from an unopposed protest during the State Opening excluded a tolerant response. Claiming that military heroes were closet homosexuals might antagonise individuals, but that was within the rules of the game governing legitimate political protest; disrupting a state occasion was not. Even if it destroyed the amicable working relationship the police had developed with 'OutRage!', this was a price worth paying.[12]

The confrontation over the State Opening of Parliament had a profound impact on the relationship between the police and OutRage! In OutRage!'s view, the police had broken an agreement, the result of which was that for the final Equality Now demonstration, the police were deceived, and not told the full extent of the action. The result was a riot.

The Equality Now March on Parliament took take place on 25 July. In theory, it was due to be a peaceful march to Parliament, assembling at Piccadilly Circus, handing in a letter of protest to Downing Street, and rallying at the Broadway at Scotland Yard. The police allowed the march to be dealt with by a chief inspector, believing it to be a small demonstration with no more than 150 marchers. However, the police noticed that in an advertisement in *Time Out*, a gathering at the Queen Victoria Memorial near Buckingham Palace was mentioned. OutRage! said they were merely going to have a 'picnic' there. The police agreed that small groups only could travel there.

We were told we would not have permission to march, we were supposed to just rush past Downing Street and disperse. We asked to have a picnic in St James's Park, all of which had been refused. Some of us were drumming, we had planned this before, to draw the whole crowd to the gates of Downing Street.

FERNANDO GUASCH

We were kissing as well. I remember Steve Cook grabbing my neck, and thinking 'Oh, I've fancied this man for years!'

KEVIN

When we got into Whitehall, we put into effect a plan to break the police lines at Downing Street and to have a sit-down.

STEVE COOK

A small group, of which I was part, broke away, because the police were trying to channel us in one lane. The traffic was able to go the other way, and that wasn't really what we'd intended to do. We wanted to hold up the traffic. So a group of us, one by one, slipped off and then we all sat in the road blocking the other side.

GRAHAM KNIGHT

The whole crowd sat down for a good half-hour. We wanted arrests. We sat there long enough to put up a soapbox, in emulation of John Major's soapbox during the election campaign, and made speeches. It was the anniversary of the '67 act, and John Beeson produced a copy of a shit-stained '67 act. I ripped it up on the soapbox.

FERNANDO GUASCH

Unusually, rather than shouting for the Prime Minster John Major, the group chanted for his opera-loving wife Norma. Although the sit-down was good-natured, the police were clearly getting worried and already calling for reinforcements.

That seemed to be all going well. The cameras were there. And then the police basically got very rough. I was pulled backwards by the arms, then leaned forward and was just dropped on my head. They weren't going to be nice. A lot of people got treated quite roughly at that point.

GRAHAM KNIGHT

Nobody knew what the fuck we were supposed to do. It was not going according to any of our plans. At one point, Peter freaked out absolutely. He came up to me and said 'I don't want to handle this.' They were making a passage for us, saying we could only leave the street in groups of one or two, and people felt very hostile. I grabbed the megaphone and tried to calm people down.

FERNANDO GUASCH

The march moved on to Parliament Square, but protestors were only allowed to travel in groups of three. From Parliament, the police attempted to disperse the crowd, although OutRage! members still hoped to make their way to St James's Park for a final rally.

The crowd went past Westminster Abbey, to the top of Victoria Street, they stopped us again and then channelled the crowd into a side street. They formed a cordon. It was at that point that people broke away, up the pavement area near St James's tube. For some reason, the police hadn't blocked off all the avenues. So groups started to free fall from down Victoria Street.

STEVE COOK

I thought it was quite dangerous. The Sisters ran into Westminster Cathedral. I remember getting caught in a back street. Somehow I got lumbered with the loudhailer for Peter who was right at the front and Nick de Marco was pushing from the back. I was face to face with this policeman who said 'You come any further and I'll arrest you' and I said, 'I don't want to come any closer!'

DAVID ARNOLD

The group then just made up its own rules. The group began to form its own opinion about what should happen and a number of leaders began to spring up. The objective became to meet at Buckingham Palace. It was at the back of our minds already. The only satisfaction we got was that the group managed to get to St James's Park and regroup.

STEVE MAYES

The March on Downing Street finally ended up in St James's Park, where Dave Arnold and the loudspeaker gave a final address, and the crowd dispersed. The action resulted in a marked change of attitude from the police, who felt they could no longer trust OutRage!, even if it was partly their own actions at the State Opening which had led to the breakdown of communications between the two parties.

At the debrief that followed... there was general regret that the leader of the group [sic] had not been arrested and that the protestors had managed to escape the containment in Caxton Street. However, it was acknowledged that the event had been peaceful. Only two arrests were made throughout the afternoon. Perhaps most importantly of all, police made it clear that the relationship between themselves and 'OutRage!' would henceforth be regarded as hostile.[13]

Equality Now was the most ambitious project that OutRage! had attempted. It involved hundreds if not thousands of lesbians and gay men, and succeeded in raising issues of lesbian and gay equality in the mainstream press and media. It left its organizers exhausted, but with stacks of photographs, props and newspaper clippings. It had also formed the Tuesday Group which would later become instrumental in changing, again, the structure and make-up of OutRage!

NOTES

1. 'Equality Now' proposal, Peter Tatchell, 24 October 1991, circulated to OutRage! members.
2. 'Equality Now' proposal.
3. 'Equality Now' proposal.
4. P.A.J. Waddington, *Liberty and Order: Public Order Policing in a Capital City* (UCL Press, 1994) p. 180. Mr Waddington followed the events covering Equality Now as part of a research programme he was conducting at the University of Reading. His book is an interesting critique of policing practice, particularly those areas regarding OutRage! and Gay Pride.
5. OutRage! legal guidelines, 'March on Parliament', 6 February 1992.
6. Waddington, *Liberty and Order*, pp. 181–2.
7. Terry Sanderson is a well-known gay journalist and agony aunt.
8. Waddington, *Liberty and Order*, p. 182.
9. Waddington, *Liberty and Order*, pp. 182–3.
10. Letter from OutRage! to Rt Hon John Major MP, Rt Hon Neil Kinnock MP, Rt Hon Paddy Ashdown MP, Mr Dafydd Wigley MP and Mr Alex Salmond MP, 5 March 1992.
11. Letter addressed to the Secretary of State for Employment, 2 April 1992.
12. Waddington, *Liberty and Order*, pp. 184–5.
13. Waddington, *Liberty and Order*, p. 190.

EIGHT

Another Night of Long Knives

The year 1992 began well for OutRage! Not only were there plans for the momentous Equality Now campaign, but there was also a welcome zap on the *Evening Standard* Awards, held on 26 January. Following a homophobic review of Derek Jarman's work by the *Standard*'s film critic Alexander Walker, and a series of anti-gay and anti-AIDS articles and reports, Jarman turned down a special award, and OutRage! marked the event by picketing outside and infiltrating the ceremony. Other award winners, notably actress Shirley MacLaine, publicly expressed support for the demonstrators, kissing and congratulating them.

The *Evening Standard* has a very long history. It's not as bad as the *Sun*. The *Evening Standard* aren't really responsible for the falling of the GLC, but were behind it.

MARTIN MAYNARD

Patrick never washed his face again because [Shirley MacLaine] kissed him!

LYNNE SUTCLIFFE

We'd done a poster campaign against the *Evening Standard* where we made up loads of posters saying 'buy your homophobia here' and we'd gone round one night at two o'clock in the morning. After great interest by everybody, three of us ended up doing it. Everyone had a passionately good idea, but when you said 'OK we'll meet at three o'clock in the morning at this place', nobody turned up! So three of us went round with this bucket of paste that had been sitting in my cupboard for three days because we weren't quite sure when we'd do it and we found loads of *Evening Standard* booths in Oxford Street, round Piccadilly and put posters up.

MEGAN RADCLIFFE

Less than a month later, OutRage! joined protests by ACT UP and the Sisters of Perpetual Indulgence against Benetton's use of a picture showing HIV-positive David Kirby dying, as part of an advertising strategy. Going into shops and trashing the displays brought much media coverage, but also criticism from other quarters that the Benetton adverts were 'art', and the campaign had been given permission to go ahead by Kirby's own family.[1]

The family of David Kirby was utterly savvy about what was happening with Benetton's use of this, and everything they predicted happened. Although Benetton were cynical and stupid, they became the vehicle for something significant.

STEVE MAYES

I also had a problem with the Benetton demos because it persecuted shop-workers. One of the good things about the left was that they'd have said 'This is picking on shop girls!'

LISA POWER

Meanwhile, OutRage! continued with some of its cruising. The setting up of LABIA had brought up the question of 'lesbian cruising' and LABIA attempted to set up its own lesbian cruising area on Hampstead Heath, which proved to be a complete disaster as far as setting up a cruising ground was concerned, but more effective in publicizing OutRage!'s safer-sex packs for women.

I remember supporting them, and Megan saying it was the same three people up there all the time. The men were laughing and saying why do you want it? I was thinking it wasn't a matter of why they wanted it: they wanted it and if other people wanted it then it should happen. Hampstead Heath always seemed this extraordinary place where you could go and find somebody cooking sausages next to somebody in SAS uniform next to somebody leaning over tree stumps. We had this idea of putting *The Bacchi* on at Hampstead Heath to try and say something about the kind of indulgence we saw and do that outdoors.

LYNNE SUTCLIFFE

Meanwhile – of course! – the gay men were cruising as ever, and attempting their own 'safer cruising' campaigns. On 29 May, they attempted a campaign on Clapham Common. The campaign was a mixture of safer-sex information and resources, and defence against queerbashings which had taken place recently on the common.

They were handing round condoms and so on, and it pelted down with rain, it absolutely pissed down. A few people huddled under trees, and this queen jumping around in a pink cagoule out of nowhere! Everyone got absolutely drenched. There were other groups doing it and it felt like OutRage! were stepping on their toes in a way.

JAMES KIERNEY

The big turning point for me, when I thought 'this isn't for me', was the queerbashing on Clapham Common. Some men had seen it and run away, and Aamir and Martin and Steve Cook thought this was wrong, and set up Queers Bash Back. I remember Aamir doing placards that, to me, advocated violence and OutRage! had always been about non-violent direct action. I can see where it's coming from, but I don't think that's the way to deal with it.

AJAY

[Queers Bash Back] was set up initially to be involved in things that OutRage! couldn't be involved in, using physical force against queer-bashers who were attacking cruisers. Some people were being beaten up at Shirley Fields at Croydon. Originally it was going to be a group within OutRage!, but it was decided we couldn't meet within OutRage! because we may use force.

DICE

'Queers Bash Back' worked much better as a slogan and an idea than as a coherent and organized group. In July, as the Royal Tournament in Earls Court was underway, the traditional threats from Army personnel to gay men on the street emerged. OutRage!, and Queers Bash Back, organized a picket of the Tournament on 8 July, and groups of men paraded round selling the familiar OutRage! whistles. The police had been told not to make arrests as a result of OutRage!'s presence, and two additional units of military police were dispatched and all military personnel had been informed that any attacks would be severely punished.

There were troops going out drunk after the tattoo and beating up gay men so we had to organize a counter-demonstration. We turned round and made the army aware of it all, and the police. We got quite a few members from that, we swept up some young queens who came along to OutRage!

MARTIN MAYNARD

Martin and I were standing outside Bromptons. We were selling whistles, and the owner came out and told us to go away because his customers didn't get queerbashed. Luckily, Martin Corbett came round the corner at that point and dealt with it very admirably.

DAVE ARNOLD

The self-defence strategy took on a more overt form when the OutRage! office received tip-offs from anti-fascists that gay pubs and clubs in Soho were about to be targeted by the British National Party, who were holding a rally in Central London. One pub, the Central Station in King's Cross, had already been the target of a CS canister attack. On 8 August, a large group of anti-fascists and OutRage! members gathered in central Soho to defend the clubs. Quite what a couple of dozen queens were supposed to do to stop rampaging fascists from attacking queer pubs was never explained, but small groups were stationed in pubs, while other 'mobile' units kept an eye out for any trouble.[2]

I spent all day organizing this thing. I said to Scotland Yard 'We'll be there in groups, but we are non-violent, and we are relying on the police to be there.' They were desperate to prove something. Some very straight people came along, like Militant. All the action was going on in Trafalgar Square. There was a weird sense of solidarity, not knowing quite what was going to happen.

MARTIN MAYNARD

Quite what I thought I was doing there I don't know, my reaction would be 'Stop!' There was me and a woman, having to stand outside the door of Village Soho. It was ridiculous! We looked at each other and thought, 'Well, what on earth are we going to do if we get attacked?' So we both agreed we'd go and have a coffee somewhere. I remember Steve Cook walking by with Aamir, and his Queers Bash Back T-shirt, and he had something wrapped around his knuckle, and I realized I'd made the right decision [to leave OutRage!].

AJAY

Chris Woods, myself, we were all wearing these Queers Bash Back T-shirts and we had skinheads' DMs on. We must have looked like fascists. Some gay men look very similar to skinheads. We ended up getting trashed in Compton's and playing pinball. We walked down to Leicester Square to get something to eat. We were in a pizza restaurant and the police brought us out of this restaurant because they thought we were the actual skinheads going round Soho.

JAMES KIERNEY

It turned out that there was a strong BNP presence in Central London that day, but the police had kept it confined and out of 'queer space'.

On 9 October, OutRage! continued its cruising actions by organizing one of its least successful zaps at Hyde Park.

The police had been harassing cruisers, and we were going into the park, but by this time it was dark and [the idea was] we would find cruisers and inform them that police were there. We got to the park, vanished into the dark and that was it! What could you do? Went in the shrubs to find queers, everyone cruised like mad and went home. It was the most monumentally pathetic action I've ever seen in my life.

STEVE MAYES

Can you hear the drums?

In May, OutRage! were made aware of a statement allegedly made by the managing director of insurance company Clerical Medical Investment, based in Bristol with registered offices in London. Following a proposal to include 'sexual orientation' in the company's equal opportunities policy, Roger Corley was alleged to have said that the company would be required to employ 'perverts, child abusers and sex offenders'. In a joint zap organized with OutRage! Bristol, the company's Bristol and London offices were hit. In London, bandit alarms were set off when a group of demonstrators infiltrated the offices. After being physically ejected, they joined a main group of noisy protestors outside sounding fog-horns and blowing whistles for half an hour before Mr Corley and his solicitor agreed to meet Fernando.

His version of the story was that they had been concerned that the inclusion of 'sexual orientation' into their equal opportunities policy might not have been tight enough to exclude child-abusers. He said that it had never been their intention to call gays and lesbians 'perverts' – he was very clearly shaken and frightened. He mentioned that they had been receiving phone calls from all over the country. Corley was anxious that this was not reported as a case of us having 'bullied them into it' and stressed that their *written* inclusion of these words in their policy document would not, as far as he was concerned, mark a change in their actual treatment of gay and lesbian employees, which he claimed had always been good. The solicitor at this point said that she had been working at the company for many years and that there was no discrimination on the grounds of sexuality.

FERNANDO GUASCH

Clerical Medical did change their policy to exclude discrimination against anyone based on their sexual orientation, and the case prompted more cases where OutRage! were asked to intervene concerning discrimination in the workplace.

Battered, bruised, bleeding

Throughout the year, OutRage! meetings were being bogged down by report-backs, factionalism and accusations of 'entryism'.[3] In particular, the Lesbian and Gay Campaign Against Racism and Fascism (LGCARF) was seen as a disruptive element and intent on using OutRage! meetings for its own ends. Given the history of other lesbian and gay organizations having gone to the wall because of sectarian politics, members of OutRage! were alarmed at what they saw as a structure which allowed for entryism.

They were putting forward very politically correct arguments but in a very disruptive and divisive way. The meetings were full of accusations, completely unfounded, malicious accusations of sexism, racism, to the point where Peter was being called fascist. It created so much acrimony, and people being driven away from the group, it was really a question of all hands on deck.

JOHN JACKSON

You'd have a vote on something or other, and people would just put their hands up for anything. Gay men are like sheep anyway, someone puts their hand up and they all put their hands up. They could be voting on anything whatsoever.

JAMES KIERNEY

It felt to me and Catherine that LGCARF were just jumping on that bandwagon. They were not getting much publicity for their own work. It felt like they were jumping on the success of OutRage! and distracted an awful lot of business away from OutRage!

MEGAN RADCLIFFE

I had a conversation with Nick de Marco [of LGCARF] and asked 'how many members have you got?', and was told in no uncertain terms that that information was privy to comrades and members of the central committee. He was coming out with all the pseudo-Marxist jargon and we got onto the Spanish Civil War and I said 'La Pasionaria' and he said 'Who's La Pasionaria?'

MARTIN MAYNARD

I remember describing them at the time as an opportunistic infection on the body politic.

DAVID ARNOLD

They started saying 'You in OutRage! need to do this…', they never spoke as part of the group. It was a long time before the OutRage! side decided to do anything about it because LGCARF were very good at playing on people's guilt, so they managed to carry along a lot of people. A lot of people just hoped it would go away.

STEVE COOK

We had to have private meetings when they weren't around to decide how to deal with them. We used to have a Tuesday meeting anyway, and during those meetings we'd set aside some time to say 'If Nick [de Marco] said this on Thursday, how would we deal with it?' or 'If Nick did that on Thursday, how were we going to deal with it?' We had to make sure that we stuck to an agenda in OutRage!, and that was a queer agenda.

NICK CAVE

We had secret meetings to try and decide how we would handle the meetings. For me, that was the start of the real problems. There was another meeting outside the group, making decisions that it would then bring to the group to rubber stamp, and agendas were already being planned in another meeting. It was very difficult to disagree with anything, because there was already a group of people who'd sorted out their line. That led to why I left.

GRAHAM KNIGHT

At the time, not only were there 'affinity groups' to look at particular actions, meet and organize them and then dissolve, but also the 'focus groups' including the newly formed YOUTH (Young radical queers Ostracizing Ubiquitous Tyrannical Heterosexism). As these groups were prioritized for a report-back at the beginning of each meeting, resentment grew as members of LGCARF were alleged to 'infiltrate' the groups and use the report-back times to prolong debates about non-queer issues. Even for members of the focus groups, things were proving difficult. In at least one meeting, things even became violent:

I had some question in mind. Nick de Marco stood up and said 'No, it's my question.' I lost my cool and said 'fucking wanker'. 'How dare you talk to me like that,' he said. 'You're a fucking wanker,' I said. Madness! Nick de Marco stands up and comes over to me and says 'Don't talk to me like that' and I said 'Fuck off you little prick' and he took a swing at me. I took a swing back. It was all macho posturing crap. Martin Harrington said I landed the first blow, and Nick de Marco then said 'Well, actually I lashed out first.' I apologized to the meeting.

DAVID ARNOLD

It wasn't easy for them, me going in, saying 'This is what we can be doing with black people, this is how you can encourage more black members.' It was difficult to be part of this group that didn't want to see you as being different. The youth group was very successful, we had a focus, but the black group didn't work at all. The black communities saw OutRage! as white, middle-class gay men, with a few women thrown in for good measure. It was frustrating to want to see it being successful but being hampered each time because there was no level of commitment from the group.

ALAN JARMAN

We were cited with wasting time in meetings when LABIA hadn't reported for over three months. We wasted money – well all the leaflets were done on my Apple Mac at work, it was all photocopied at my workplace. We hardly asked for any money at all. We did ask for some around Jennifer Saunders. Where was the wastage there? It felt like we were being pushed out because they couldn't be bothered – 'Just go away, just leave us alone, because we've got bigger and better and more important things to do.'

MEGAN RADCLIFFE

There was one point where we saw a way out. I remember trying to analyse the structural politics of the group, and I presented a plan at this meeting in the pub where we could kill two birds with one stone. From an anarchist point of view – which seemed a one-up from a Trotskyite point of view – what brought me to OutRage! was the excitement of open meetings, where nobody had privilege, and you should get rid of the structural parts of the group that allowed certain individuals, certain factions, a privilege. We called a meeting on a Thursday when we knew LGCARF were off demonstrating against fascism in Europe, and we called all the founding fathers. A couple of people presented a proposal that we should return to OutRage!'s non-hierarchical structure.

STEVE COOK

I went up to Housmans and tracked down their magazine. They were LGCARF, which was the sister organization of the Campaign Against Racism and Fascism, which was a broad front organization set up by the

Revolutionary Internationalist League, which is the British contingent of the International Trotskyist Committee for the Political Regeneration of The Fourth International, which is Nick de Marco and a couple of mates. I found a couple of articles in their magazine – 'LGCARF have gone along to OutRage! to show them the right road to revolution and are being rejected by bourgeois capitalist hacks' – and I handed that round at the meeting.

MARTIN MAYNARD

I argued against the response then, and I still disagree with it. I don't know how else we could have done it, but as an open group, we had to allow dissent. You have to allow other voices.

GRAHAM KNIGHT

I think they were probably right to abolish the focus groups. I don't think they were dissolved in the right way because people weren't there and felt deeply betrayed and hurt and let down. I voted for them going that day.

LYNNE SUTCLIFFE

In the end, OutRage! quite rightly said this is causing us problems, therefore we'll abolish the focus groups, which was seen as an antagonistic statement against special interests. It was purely an act of self-preservation. It was one of those moments where OutRage! reinvented itself. There was a change of personnel in the process. What's held OutRage! together again and again has been this focus on fighting homophobia.

STEVE MAYES

The meeting of 25 June proved to be a watershed for OutRage! A long discussion of focus groups and their purpose ensued, echoing arguments two years previously about OutRage!'s future and direction. Peter Tatchell proposed dissolving all existing affinity, focus and caucus groups except the two admin groups QUID and QUANGO and in future to set groups up only to organize particular actions according to OutRage!'s constitution. The motion was amended not to re-discuss this issue within 12 months, and to reaffirm OutRage!'s existing constitution, emphasizing the power of vibewatchers to make sure speakers stick to OutRage!'s constitution. Of the 41 people in attendance, there was only one abstention and three votes against the motion.

I was absolutely fuming. How dare they! We were really lucky that Catherine just happened to be there that night. Catherine came round afterwards and said 'You won't believe what's happened, they've just abolished the group.' And I said, 'Well, isn't that unconstitutional?' We were called focus groups because we were supposed to be permanent. However long OutRage! was going, apparently that's how long we were going. I eventually secured the minutes, after writing to OutRage! and almost being abused. Now there are some comments in there about we're making people feel guilty – then we were doing our job. That's what we were set up to do, to make you realize 'Hey, there are other people in this group, that are putting time, effort, money, whatever, in.'

MEGAN RADCLIFFE

We got into trouble immediately. Some journalist from the *Pink Paper* ran this and interviewed Megan, who hadn't been at the vote, and Ajay and Tony and LGCARF, and concocted this whole article such that a right-wing gang of OutRage! had excluded women, black and disabled people. The next meeting was very unpleasant because LGCARF, all the people who hadn't been there, people like Keith Alcorn and Chris Woods, turned up in their journalist capacity. LGCARF were challenging the resolution at every point. There were two or three meetings where we were made to behave like fascist dictators and 'vibewatch! vibewatch! vibewatch!' every time somebody opened their mouths.

STEVE COOK

We fired off a letter to the *Pink* and it had a ripple. OutRage! wrote back and gave their reasons. It just felt like bullshit. I think they realized they'd shot themselves in the foot, but there was nothing they could do. I could be wrong, but I think they realized they made a mistake and ever since then they've been in denial about the whole thing. I did my two pennies' worth and I don't want that to be lost. It's about the fact that I wanted to do something for the people who helped me when I first came out, who are still being persecuted. I've known too many people who've been affected, been abused, to want to stop doing that.

MEGAN RADCLIFFE

I think that really changed OutRage! It became very defensive. Vibewatchers were there to silence people, they weren't there to keep good vibes, they were there for 'You can't say that!' or 'You can't talk about that!'. It got us a very bad feedback from the press, who didn't really understand the motives. I think the motives were good motives.

GRAHAM KNIGHT

They hadn't managed to take OutRage! over, but they had managed to cripple it in terms of its PR. If we hadn't got rid of the caucus groups, I don't think we'd have got through that summer. The meetings were no longer this exchange of fiery ideology. We ended up with a group of people who shared a very clear vision, a very explicit agenda, which was fighting homophobia. We evolved at that point into something which doesn't have a counterpart.

STEVE COOK

If we had not gone through that period in the wilderness, to reassess our strength, to reassess our motivation, we could never have developed the confidence to then go on and to brave the Jakobovits thing. We then went on and were able to brave accusations of anything.

FERNANDO GUASCH

NOTES

1 Along with other Sisters of Perpetual Indulgence, I attended many of the protests against Benetton. One of my most moving memories of the Benetton demos was picketing the Carnaby Street shop and handing out leaflets to passers-by, explaining the nature of the action. Unnervingly, a group of skinheads stood drinking and watching us, occasionally making comments that we failed to hear. Feeling a little brave (or stupid) I decided to approach them, wearing my nun's habit, and explain the action; the guy I spoke to listened quietly as I talked about the David Kirby picture, how we felt it to be cold and calculating to use AIDS as an issue to sell jumpers. At the end, he shook my hand and said 'Good for you; my Dad died of AIDS.' He hadn't discussed it with anyone before.
2 Through some bizarre logic, my flatmate Adam Jeanes and I were left to 'protect' Compton's in Soho from any trouble. Neither of us were bouncer material. We had nothing to defend ourselves with apart from a can of glitter hairspray I'd brought with me – the idea being that they'd get a jolly nasty shine if they came anywhere near us. We had some sort of plan to run screaming into the toilets if anyone came near us. It did feel very much like a *Carry On* film or Julian and Sandy sketch – 'Bona Bodyguards'. We ended up getting pissed at the bar.
3 Entryism was a common practice whereby far left groups attempted to dominate and control the agenda of gay activism.

NINE

'Sister, Sister, It's an Outrage!'

In July 1992, the Congregation for the Doctrine of the Faith, the Vatican's doctrinal watchdog, issued a document which attempted to help its bishops deal with the thorny issue of anti-discrimination legislation, particularly in America. The document referred to homosexuality as an 'objective disorder' and claimed that 'There are areas in which it is not unjust discrimination to take sexual orientation into account – for example, in the placement of children for adoption or foster care, in employment of teachers or athletic coaches and in military recruitment.'[1]

In a swift rebuttal of the statement, OutRage! wrote to Cardinal Basil Hume complaining that such pronouncements 'give theological legitimacy to anti-gay prejudice and actively encourage the victimisation of lesbians and gay men'.[2] The letter went on to ask Cardinal Hume if 'you personally endorse the Vatican's statements? Will the Catholic Church in the UK in future oppose legislation for lesbian and gay human rights?' A reply from his office announced that Cardinal Hume had a long series of visits and engagements and would be in contact in the future.

I went along to a meeting at Steve Cook's house the night before. I got nominated by Peter to be the one doing the main interviewing. We met at Wimbledon tube station and it was just after that woman was killed on Wimbledon Common, so there were a lot of police around. I was quite nervous.

MARTIN MAYNARD

The ruse was arranged that we would pose as a student newspaper and would talk to him [the Vatican's Ambassador to Britain] then gain access into the [Vatican Embassy]. It worked brilliantly. We had a back-up group of a dozen or so, armed with placards and cameras and all the rest. They all hid in shrubs outside the building, in dribs and drabs positioned themselves as four of us went in by invitation and awaited the arrival of the Papal Nuncio. He arrived and his first words were 'Ah, what a nice group of young men!'

STEVE MAYES

I was having to maintain this conversation with one of the highest dignitaries of the Catholic Church in this country, knowing that Peter and co. were just about to come through the door.

MARTIN MAYNARD

My role in all of this was as photographer, to find a location for the Nuncio's photograph. So I said, 'While you're talking I'll just find a suitable location where I can take your picture.' So I retraced my steps, fortunately not being tracked by nuns or anything, and managed to secure the entrance. I gave the signal, the shrubs erupted and everyone charged through the front door which I was obligingly holding open for them.

STEVE MAYES

We were hogging around by the bus stop. I saw a police car go by, and thought they knew about it already. I remember getting in there, the Papal Nuncio attacking Peter.

DICE

He was horrified, sitting there having this pleasant interview with people admiring him, and suddenly this room was full of nasty people being very rude to him. He stood there blinking in utter disbelief, probably thinking he was going to be assassinated or something. We said, this is a non-violent demonstration, blah blah blah. It slowly dawned on him that he was surrounded by queers, as all these posters came out, and the cameras started flashing, and he rushed to the door with his finger in the air, and the words on his lips were 'Sister, sister, this is an outrage!' which of course was dead right.

STEVE MAYES

He'd only recently been raised to diplomatic status. He's protected by the Diplomatic Response Unit. We had to scramble out, and it was one of those gravel drives, it was like you see getaways in the movies – he switched the engine on and the wheels went and didn't catch.

MARTIN MAYNARD

Peter went in disguise, he wore dark glasses, but they saw through that, they managed to identify him in the photographs. He and one or two others were interviewed by the police, who were asking him for names, addresses. They wanted to pursue a conspiracy charge, which was very serious and essentially they refused to cooperate. The nuncio did his utmost to have the whole thing prosecuted and pursued in any form he could.

STEVE MAYES

The zap on the Vatican Embassy got enormous coverage in the press, and was almost treated as a 'diplomatic incident' although the case was never taken further, possibly because before fleeing to the kitchen the Papal Nuncio, Archbishop Luigi Barbarito, had forcefully knocked Peter to the floor. Photographs in the press that week showed a dumbfounded nuncio surrounded by placards saying 'Stop Crucifying Queers', 'Vatican Prejudice Stirs Anti Gay Hate' and 'Stop Papal Bull!'

On Sunday 9 August, OutRage! planned another zap, this time during a service at Westminster Cathedral. While some members picketed outside the 11 o'clock service, others, infiltrated the church itself.[3]

Twenty people turned up, sat themselves down in the congregation, took part in the service and just before the sermon, Martin Harrington went up to the front and said the usual, 'Don't be alarmed…' Then everyone went up with him, unfurled their placards, stood in a row at the front of the Cathedral.

Peter had written an alternative sermon, and he started reading it, and he got a good couple of minutes in stunned silence, with this wonderful tableau of everyone standing there with placards, and then the organist started up. So we started blowing whistles and proceeded down the aisle with Peter sermonizing. There was an attempted assault on Peter, some creepy little Catholic man came into the aisle, genuflected, and then tried to rip Peter's placard away. We got all the way to the doors before the police arrived.

STEVE COOK

I was walking down the aisle shouting and I remember that when it was reported, I was called 'Miss Throaty' because they thought I had a deep voice. It was one of my first 'handbag' times – we churched up and had straight drag, and I had this handbag that I used to take, which was terribly kind of formidable and was brilliant for concealing props and whistles and posters.

LYNNE SUTCLIFFE

For the next demonstration against the Catholic Church, OutRage! decided to turn up the heat and adopt a more openly confrontational style. The second demonstration at Westminster Cathedral, on Sunday 20 September, was advertised as uncompromisingly angry:

> **HOLY SHIT!**
>
> **TEACHING?**
> **ADOPTION?**
> **FOSTER CARE?**
> **COUNCIL HOUSING?**
> **CIVIL RIGHTS?**
> **THE VATICAN SAYS FORGET IT!!!**
>
> THEY SAY THERE IS A MORAL OBLIGATION TO DISCRIMINATE AGAINST QUEERS – HOMOSEXUALITY IS AN OBJECTIVE DISORDER – IF WE FIGHT FOR OUR RIGHTS WE BRING VIOLENCE UPON OURSELVES.
>
> **WE SAY FUCK YOU!!!**
>
> JOIN THE OUTRAGE! QUEER CRUCIFIXION AND STOP THEIR PAPAL BULLSHIT[4]

The plan to 'crucify' a lesbian immediately got a refusal from the police, who banned anything that might be seen as 'blasphemous'. Nevertheless, plans went ahead to construct an eight-foot-high crucifix.

The Friday, I was press releasing and I picked the short straw, I think the *Catholic Herald* or the *Universe*. 'Can I interest you in this story?' and the guy went 'Making fun of the greatest occurrence in the history of the universe!' and it was a case of 'No, the resurrection is that. OutRage! are not telling you the ins and outs of Catholic theology, but...' He put the phone down.

MARTIN MAYNARD

We had a banner, a 60-foot banner that we had spent hundreds of pounds on. We had tried it out, and just by pulling a piece of rope the whole thing would have unfurled and covered the whole thing. But for some reason, the police knew we were coming and they had not been able to put it up. So when we arrived, we were already very pissed off.

FERNANDO GUASCH

We were bringing the crucifix out and the police dropped on us, and I remember having a tug of war with the crucifix going backwards and forwards, nuns and all. The police struggled, got it on the floor, and then stood on it to stop us moving it. Quite a funny sight!

NICK CAVE

The cross was confiscated by the police very violently. There's this picture of the police standing on the cross, which given they were there to prevent a blasphemy was just outrageous, a shocking piece of irony, trampling on the cross.

STEVE MAYES

I was just standing there at the time, and suddenly this policeman and woman whirled on me and said 'Right, you're nicked mate' and I was led off to the police van.

DAVID ARNOLD

Although unable to crucify a gay man in front of the Cathedral, wearing an OutRage! 'Queer to Eternity' T-shirt, David Arnold was later supported by two Sisters of Perpetual Indulgence as he was carried prone, arms outstretched, to the Cathedral. An alternative sermon was staged in front of the Cathedral. The behaviour of the police led to a formal complaint, after four arrests. In a five-page letter detailing the incidents, OutRage! complained that police had used unnecessary force and shouted homophobic comments such as 'Fuck off' and 'Piss off you fucking queer.'

The experience taught OutRage! to be more systematic about its actions, and a sharpening of manoeuvres and stage management resulted. A repeat confrontation with Westminster Cathedral and this time Cardinal Hume himself took place on Palm Sunday, during the Bishop's procession at Westminster Cathedral on 9 April 1993. The Palm Day procession was a high-profile media event, and during it OutRage! were being filmed for a programme on volunteering, *The V Word*, for Channel 4, presented by Margi Clarke.

Having being brought up a Catholic, I felt I'd been damaged by the Church, I'd spent years trying to be 'straight', praying, and going through hell in my teenage years. I felt angry with the Church when I began to realize that it was OK to be queer, and that it was just a part of me, something that wouldn't change no matter how much you prayed. A number of teenagers who commit suicide each year go through that trouble. I took great pride in the actions against the Catholic Church. There was a procession coming through the piazza, there were a number of priests and monks, Cardinal Hume himself at the front, throwing palms. As they came round we passed among them shouting things like 'Church of hatred, church of fear, stop crucifying queers!'

DICE

I had to yawn and stretch when I saw them coming round the corner which was a signal to someone else to phone the people in the van. The van drove up, it was very slickly done, Martin and John Beeson had worked out the choreography of who was putting down which strut. It was a lesbian [being crucified] this time, which was good. There were a lot of sisters there who made a tableau round the cross. We had some brilliant conversations with people. There were some men from America, older gays, who came out to see what we were doing.

LYNNE SUTCLIFFE

There was an Irishman and I was saying I'd been brought up Catholic, and this guy said 'I don't go to Mass to pray to the Pope, I go to Mass to pray to God. What the Pope says is wrong.'

DICE

After the Palm Sunday procession, every night in Holy Week some of us went back and held a very dignified vigil outside in the Piazza. [Cardinal Hume] did produce a public document, you'd have to be a theologian to have found anything in it that was great news, although Peter did claim to have interpreted it. We then kind of lost interest in it. We'd got this frustrating, intellectual quibbling around semantics in this correspondence. We'd done everything outrageous in terms of debating the issue.

STEVE COOK

Porn again

The man connected with new anti-pornography campaigns which had caused problems for gay porn and literature, and had also spent an estimated £3 million on Operation Spanner under the guise of it breaking a large-scale vice ring, was Superintendent Michael Hames, the Head of the Obscene Publications Squad. Hames had spoken repeatedly at the National Viewers' and Listeners' Association, a political platform for censorship crusaders, and Hames's officers had also given evidence to the Isle of Man Parliament to support their legislation against homosexuality.

When OutRage! learned that Hames was due to address the National Women's Council censorship meeting on 'Liberty or Licence' on 21 September 1992, it seemed too good an opportunity to miss. Publicity for the OutRage! action emphasized that 'This is not just about pornography, but the obscene abuse of power.' On the day of the event, flyers given out to attendees directly challenged Supt Hames and the Obscene Publications Squad:

Why are you here? Why does a public servant spend so much time and resources on public platforms talking pure politics – at such a high cost to the tax payer? Why did you comment on Hampstead Heath being 'colonized by gays'? You are establishing yourself as a policeman of morality – not of the law. Were you really looking for obscene publications in the shrubbery? How can you justify your complicity with the Manx government in their attempts to maintain their illegal legislation (in flagrant breach of European community laws on homosexuality)?[5]

We all went along in straight drag. There was one very intelligent and liberal Pakistani or Indian psychiatrist there. I stood up in my right-wing Tory aspect and said 'Are you going to suggest that if we had gentle loving porn, we'd be a better culture as a consequence?' And he basically said yes! The audience were rather flummoxed at that. It was all going swimmingly and then Hames comes on. Fernando gets up, walks to the front, cool as a cucumber, grabs the microphone and all hell breaks loose, whistles, foghorns. The security guard was chasing people round. They cleared that out the way and another group of people stood up, and then a third group. A woman next to me said 'These homosexuals aren't doing themselves any good with this sort of behaviour.' And then I stood up. 'Oh no, not you too!' After the meeting, Fernando was 'PC'd', sorry 'vibewatched', at the meeting for describing them as being 'vicious old bats'.

DAVID ARNOLD

Daring to speak love's name

Despite – or because of – OutRage!'s public confrontations with Christianity, the group was invited to help launch a book of lesbian and gay prayers. Dr Elizabeth Stuart's book, *Daring to Speak Love's Name*, had been dropped by its original publisher, the Society for Promotion of Christian Knowledge (SPCK), and taken up eventually by mainstream publishing house Hamish Hamilton. OutRage! were invited to produce a theatrical set-piece for the launch, and elaborate plans were drawn up which included large banners, crosses, fog machines.

I was liaising with the publishing company. Someone from the *Pink Paper* phoned them and said 'Are you aware that OutRage! is contemplating an action against you and you will have male nuns pulling books from the shelves?' [The launch] was in Westminster Central Hall and the queen who was the manager of the Central Hall was the son of someone terribly powerful in the Methodist Church and had done this without really informing anyone. There was then an article in the *Sun* or the *Star* the day before, 'Gay nuns marrying one another off a stage'. There was mayhem. We weren't allowed the Stop Crucifying Queers banner, we weren't allowed to have the fog.

MARTIN MAYNARD

The controversy over OutRage!'s presence meant that the publishers made radical – and to many unacceptable – changes to OutRage!'s presentation. Taking up the theme of censorship, one OutRage! member made a speech while others stood gagged. For those who hadn't known about the change of plan, there was a lot of anger, bitterness and resentment.

Ed got up and read this prearranged statement which we democratically cobbled together beforehand and the chief guy from the publishers leapt up and grabbed the podium and said 'This is totally untrue.' I remember seeing Fernando chasing someone round the hall, digging someone in the elbows and saying 'That's why the Spanish Civil War started !'

MARTIN MAYNARD

Royal Mail failing to deliver

Because of its high profile, OutRage! often attracted people who wanted their causes taken up. Although it was difficult for OutRage! to enter into individual cases, occasionally a case illustrating larger aspects of workplace homophobia would come to light, and OutRage! felt duty-bound to intervene. One such case was the plight of postal worker Steven Watts. Watts had been suffering homophobic abuse at work, which began with jokes about him attending Freddie Mercury's funeral, and then toilet and workplace graffiti. Although he had complained to his superiors, and to his trade union, no action had been taken against the men abusing him.

The easiest solution they could find was to tell Steven to shut up, and to let the harassers off. We took it on, partly to support Steve personally but also to take on one of the country's biggest employers and educate them into how they should treat this kind of issue.

STEVE MAYES

OutRage! decided initially to send a letter to Cambridge HQ demanding that they investigate the Watts case, and then carried out a zap on the Royal Mail's London Headquarters at Old Street on 9 November 1992. Three OutRage! members went in to meet with the Head of Equal Opportunities, and the foyer was taken over with fog-horns and whistles, while a fourth member of OutRage! made it right up to the fourth floor with a blaring fog-horn. After a meeting the following Wednesday with Watts's personnel manager, it became clear that the Post Office were not taking Watts's claims of harassment seriously. OutRage! decided to take its complaints directly to Cambridge, and descended on the Post Office there on 10 December.

That was more successful, it was very easy, there were stairs, we had a plan as to exactly where we should go. We went upstairs and into the offices.

DICE

Rob Archer invented the stunningly brilliant action idea of phoning the local radio station from the midst of the action – 'Get me on air, I am speaking to you from the heart of the Post Office', to the sound of shrieks and fog-horns.

STEVE MAYES

OutRage! continued to point to the fact that the Royal Mail had its own equal opportunities policy, which it was not implementing in the Watts case. Once again, OutRage decided to flex its muscles, resulting in a historic result from one of the country's biggest employers.

We eventually went down to the Head Office in Old Street, occupied the building there and went to see the Chairperson, who was out at the time. We made our mark in such a strong way that they had to take notice. In a shot the situation was resolved. The disciplinary procedure was reviewed, Steve secured his position, his abusers were removed. We educated a major employer into how to handle homophobic abuse.

STEVE MAYES

Watts's victory was even more important because of the Royal Mail's role as one of the country's major employers, and the precedent it set in actively implementing equal opportunities policies with regard to sexuality. It was a major attack on the victimization of lesbian or gay workers, and the idea that homophobic bullying was acceptable in the workplace, or that the easiest way to deal with it was to ignore or blame the victim.

NOTES

1. Cited in the *Guardian*, 'Gays angry as Vatican backs bias', 24 July 1992.
2. OutRage! letter to Cardinal Basil Hume, 28 July 1992.
3. I attended the picket with some other Sisters of Perpetual Indulgence. Dressed in habit, we had to wait for ages while the action inside was waiting to take place. I wandered over to one of the benches in the grounds of the Cathedral and sat down. Next to me was a sweet little old lady, who smiled and confided that she'd heard about our demo on the radio that morning and wanted to come down to see what was going on. We chatted for a while about the Catholic view on homosexuality, and she told me she couldn't see what all the fuss was about. As we talked, nun to lady, a young man approached me with a leaflet. He gave me and my new friend an evangelical Christian tract, and began to ask me questions about whether I had been saved or recognized Jesus as my Lord. All of a sudden, the little old lady became perturbed at his haranguing and started telling him to leave me alone and that he should mind his own business. They started having a row about theology, with the lady refusing to answer the guy's repeated questions about what her faith was. Eventually, she shooed him off, and confided in me that she was in fact a practising Catholic and a member of the congregation at Westminster Cathedral, that she was going inside to say some prayers, and would say one for me. We said cheerio, and she wandered into the Cathedral after offering OutRage! her personal support.
4. OutRage! flyer, 'Holy Shit!', September 1992.
5. OutRage! flyer, 21 September 1992.

TEN

Music, Cameras, Action!

OutRage!, sassy media queens as they were, were also aware of the effect of the media on people's lives. Art and politics, as far as OutRage! were concerned, did and should mix. OutRage! attempted to challenge not only institutions, but also the mechanisms by which culture recreated itself.

In 1992 rock group Guns 'N' Roses became the centre for OutRage!'s wrath as a result of their homophobic lyrics, attacking women, black people and those living with AIDS. Some years earlier, Michelangelo Signorile had attacked the band's manager, David Geffen, in his column in the American pro-outing *Outweek*.

GEFFEN, YOU PIG, WE DEMAND THAT YOU IMMEDIATELY STAND UP FOR YOURSELF AND THIS COMMUNITY AND DENOUNCE AND DROP GUNS 'N' ROSES. We demand an apology for their gross, violence inciting statements – both from you for not saying anything as they spewed such venom and from them for their ignorance.[1]

A series of stickers – 'Queers say Fuck U! Guns N Roses', 'Women say Fuck U! Guns N Roses', 'Blacks say Fuck U Guns N Roses' and 'People with AIDS say Fuck U! Guns N Roses' – were produced and zaps in prominent record stores raised the issue in the music and mainstream press. On 11 April 1992, 1500 protest stickers were plastered over the band's merchandise at Tower Records in Piccadilly Circus, while staff gave a round of applause and wore stickers themselves. The action was reported in the *Sun*, *Melody Maker* and on IRN. One OutRage! member, Aamir, was arrested and charged with threatening behaviour, although the case was later dropped. A similar action occurred the following week at the Virgin Megastore. OutRage! and ACT UP also campaigned (unsuccessfully) to have Guns 'N' Roses removed from the Freddie Mercury Tribute concert, where they had been asked to play.

By May, OutRage! had found a new target. The Hollywood film *Basic Instinct*, starring Michael Douglas and Sharon Stone, had already been the target of American queer activism even before it had been released. Following the controversy surrounding *Silence of the Lambs*, criticized for its portrayal of homosexuality, Hollywood was under intense scrutiny over its representations of lesbians and gay men. As *Basic Instinct* was being shot in San Francisco, protests against its portrayal of lesbian or bisexual women as ice-pick murderers resulted in the set being closed down. The protests went on for weeks. When the film opened in America, activists picketed cinemas with posters saying 'Catherine did it', giving away the film's surprise ending.

OutRage!'s more muted response centred on the opening of *Basic Instinct*, involving a picket of the film on 8 May. Stickers attacking the film and the stars were produced.

It wasn't so much the film itself, it was the fact that it was one of Hollywood's perpetual treatments of lesbian and gays as being strange, remarkable, murderous, somehow mentally ill. We stood outside the cinema when it was being shown.

ROB KEMP

Basic Instinct came and went, but the real arguments about representations of lesbians and gay men continued. Not just Hollywood, but the music and media industries were attacked by queer activists here and in America for contributing to rather than challenging homophobia.

Although the action against Guns 'N' Roses had been fairly clear-cut, a similar action against black reggae star Buju Banton was more complicated. Banton's record *Boom-Bye-Bye* contained lyrics encouraging the killing of 'batty-boys', slang for homosexuals. OutRage! wanted to raise the issue of prosecution for inciting hatred, although this was opposed by black gay groups on the grounds that state intervention against black artists would be seen as insensitive, and cooperating with State racism. A group dedicated against homophobia within the black communities and media, Let's Rap, worked with OutRage! to raise the issue within black communities. A flurry of letters went back and forth between OutRage! and Banton's record label, Jet Star. The issue became a major story in the black and music press, and resulted in Banton being dropped from the prestigious WOMAD festival in 1992. Banton's concert at the Hammersmith Palais was leafleted by OutRage! members and members of Let's Rap on 8 December.

[It] was different from other reggae records which said 'Oh, it's nasty, we don't like it.' It was a real call for murder, in a sense. We got onto the distributors... they agreed in the end they wouldn't put the record on any compilation albums, and they wouldn't re-release it. We went round to all the major record stores and asked them not to stock it. They agreed. We called up the radio stations and asked them not to play it. In effect, what we attempted to do was get the record blocked. Whether it's the correct strategy, I'm still having doubts about. In America, they said 'Play the record, but put this statement on afterwards, saying it invites violence against gay people.' That allows the record to be heard, and keeps the debate open.

GRAHAM KNIGHT

I don't care what anyone tells you. I was living in Brixton for two and a half years and that record legitimized a lot of the homophobia amongst white and black. The number of times I was called 'batty man', and that was a phrase unheard of, virtually unheard of, until that record.

JOHN JACKSON

The general thing which everybody said was that you had to understand it in some kind of code, not really meaning kill gay men, and we didn't understand it because we weren't part of Jamaican culture. The black people who were involved didn't agree with that interpretation of it. He never apologized for it, he never made any statement at all.

GRAHAM KNIGHT

I remember writing a letter, eight or nine months down the line, about Buju giving money to a charity for children with AIDS in his own country, and had nothing to do with gay men. Somebody had been quoted and they twisted it, and said that OutRage! had forgiven Buju. I wrote in and said 'What are you talking about, no we haven't, and if this man wants to be forgiven, all he'd have to do is come out and say homophobia and bigotry are wrong' – which he hasn't.

JOHN JACKSON

Arguments about Buju, reggae and homophobia continued, and began to involve other reggae stars such as Tippa Irie and Shabba Ranks. Tippa Irie, due to attend an open meeting with the black community to discuss the issue of homophobia and reggae music, failed to show. Shabba Ranks, in an interview on TV show *The Word*, aired his conviction that gays should be crucified. OutRage! added its voice to growing criticism of Ranks, claiming that he was inciting violence, and that where he was given a public platform, those responsible were also encouraging murder of lesbians and gay men. When Shabba was invited to appear on *Top of the Pops*, OutRage! invaded Broadcasting House in Oxford Circus on 26 March.

It was the night of the Spanner demo. And a contingent went from there up to Portland Place and went into the foyer. Peter Tatchell insisted on trying to make a speech, and making a photo opportunity out of arguing with the receptionist.

STEVE COOK

A more controversial action was to follow, when it was proposed that OutRage! zap the phone-lines for the BBC's popular crime investigation programme, *Crimewatch*.

We said to *Top of the Pops* 'Show Shabba Ranks, but then show a statement saying we do not support violence against lesbians and gays.' *Top of the Pops* hadn't done it, so we thought 'Right! The real criminals are the BBC for promoting people who promote violence against lesbian and gay people.' So, we aimed to get as many people as possible to phone up *Crimewatch* while it was on to block the phone lines. That was controversial, because people said 'What about people who can't report real crimes because you're blocking the lines!' – as if phoning *Crimewatch* is the only way to report crimes!

GRAHAM KNIGHT

We went to King's Cross station. It's not there now, but at the time, there was a little hallway that had 20 to 25 BT phones, and also phones outside. We'd got a large number of phone cards, and we went up to block the phone lines of *Crimewatch*.

DICE

We phoned *Crimewatch*, said we wished to make a complaint. 'We wish to record a crime', and some of them said, 'Thank you very much' and other people were less patient with us. The programme presented the view that nothing was happening, everything was going on as usual. We felt we'd failed in a sense, but then we had information saying there'd hardly been any phone calls coming in because we blocked the phone lines.

GRAHAM KNIGHT

Fernando phoned home and his phone was engaged for ages and ages. He was by himself, yet his phone was engaged…

LYNNE SUTCLIFFE

While we were phoning, there was a guy standing there with a newspaper and we heard him talking to his mate, a plain clothes policeman, telling him where we were and what we were doing. So, a few of us said 'Here's a plain clothes policeman on the phone everybody!' He moved off, and we followed him round the tube station, trying to intimidate him and keep an eye on him.

GRAHAM KNIGHT

A further attempt to infiltrate the BBC building was made on 22 April, this time more successfully.

We walked straight past the commissionaires, who had an extremely delayed reaction, such that eight or nine of us got through, dispersed, running up as many flights of stairs as we could. Gradually some of us met each other in corridors. I remember going through the restaurant with a foghorn shouting something, and we were trying to find the newsroom. We got into the Director General's room off the boardroom and plastered it with posters, and we did get a good photograph of the clock above the Chairman of the BBC's seat with a poster – 'BBC incites hatred'. On the news programmes, they denied we'd entered the building. The police dragged everybody out and blockaded the building.

STEVE COOK

Although there was one arrest (for obstruction) the charge was dropped. A couple of days later, OutRage! also picketed the Royal Television Society's annual meeting. However, by this time a new factor was beginning to emerge in OutRage!'s criticism of the BBC. Following an article on the BBC's new equality provision paper *Extending Choice Charter*, OutRage! began a lengthy correspondence with the BBC over its lack of inclusion of lesbian and gay issues.

This was all just something sparked by my reading an article in the newspaper and taking it up in the guise of a member of OutRage! It seems to me that that was the key to OutRage!'s success – it was a group of individuals often working together, but more often lending a group's name to an individual's passion for a particular issue.

ROB KEMP

The BBC charter mentioned sexuality once and lesbians and gay men also once, in 53 pages attempting to ensure that output was broad-based and relevant to all sections of the community. A flurry of letters in April and May were given increased importance in the light of the BBC's failure to cover on any news bulletins the March on Washington for lesbian, gay and bisexual equality and civil rights, the largest-ever such march, involving over a million people. Eventually, the BBC agreed to meet with Sarah Graham, Rob Kemp and Peter Tatchell on 7 June.

The people at the meeting were Sandra Horne, Chief Personnel Officer; Kate Pluck, Equal Opportunities Officer; Jenny Abramski, Editor of Radio News; Chris Graham, No. 2 in TV Daily News; Samir Shah, Editor of Weekly and Special Programmes, TV and Richard Ayre, the Controller of Editorial Policy. Our main points were that same-sex partners should count as relatives; that people with HIV/AIDS must have protection from discrimination and be allowed flexibility at work; that anti-homophobia training should be introduced and that the Charter should specifically include lesbians and gay men at every point. We fought hard to try and make them see that lesbian and gay rights are human rights. However, they wouldn't suggest or accept possible steps to bring balance to their output.

ROB KEMP

The news agenda is almost certain to continue to rate newsworthiness in strictly heterosexual terms. They produced no justification for not covering the March on Washington except to say that the biggest human-rights march in history wasn't news. Now, they said, is queer-bashing news? – because it has been going on for years.

FERNANDO GUASCH

They heard us talk about the issues that matter to us. We told them how we think the BBC can improve its broadcasting. They said they would go away and think about the fact that the BBC has an overwhelmingly heterosexual agenda, but only time will show how successful the meeting was in educating them and producing long-term improvement.

SARAH GRAHAM

My body is beautiful

Following ongoing research as a result of the work with the 'ex-gay' cults in the UK, information was given to OutRage! regarding an 'open day' for parents of lesbians and gays, run by the Living Waters group.

The idea was to bring parents along to teach them how to handle their kids. We posed as parents and went along.

STEVE MAYES

We joined in the start of the service. It was quite tense, because there were some people there who were gesticulating madly with their hands, and gesturing that they were receiving the Word, very intense looks on their faces, all these children hanging around as well.

DICE

I remember Steve Cook pogoing to the hymns. When the sermon came, Fernando asked a question and we all blew whistles. Their response was, 'Would you like a biscuit?' and you felt like saying 'No, I'm demonstrating here, I don't want a biscuit!'

GRAHAM KNIGHT

Everyone kept coming to me and saying why are they doing such things? Why are they letting stink bombs off? I was standing there in my placatory role as usual trying to explain.

BETH LANE

We discovered a number of parents were unaware of the nature of the group and were very perturbed with some of the tactics that this brainwashing group were applying. We discovered one or two people who had very unhappy experiences who came and confessed to us. There was one Christian there who confided that he took the cure by day and went cruising by night. They knew themselves they were up against wrong thinking.

STEVE MAYES

One guy stood up and dropped his pants and showed his willy and said 'My body is beautiful, it's not dirty!' [I remember] outside having a big argument with him about how could we show our willies when there were children around! We lost that guy.

GRAHAM KNIGHT

The carnival (is over)

Aware of a burgeoning gay commercial scene, particularly in Soho around Old Compton Street, and the emergence of major new venues such as Village Soho, OutRage! decided to mobilize this energy and planned a community carnival.

Peter wanted to do an age of consent event, Queer Eros, lots of teenagers looking pretty, and we'd have a party in Piccadilly Circus. Some people turned this round and we decided to bring it in to Queer Town.

STEVE COOK

I remember talking with Martin and Aamir about putting up a sign that said 'Queer Street', months before. Peter wanted a big Valentine's card to present to Downing Street. The police were refusing to give us the street. We got signatures from every single shop in the street, we got a route, we got a samba band, and I happened to bump into The Well Oiled Sisters, who were delighted to perform. In those days, we had no money to place adverts in the press, so we'd have to give out thousands of flyers.

FERNANDO GUASCH

That was one of the best queer events I've ever been to. It was wonderful, it was very colourful, it was a mixture of politics and fun, supported by all the bars. I'm sure it was illegal, because we were on the back of this truck and we were having to hold speaker systems and stuff, otherwise they'd topple. The float was decorated very well by Martin Corbett and John Beeson.

DICE

Part of the model was the Chinese New Year celebrations, where the dragon goes and blesses the statues. We had Debbie dressed up as a dyke cupid and Mark as a male cupid, and they went to The Edge and blessed the place. The Edge was new and paid for all these pink balloons.

FERNANDO GUASCH

I remember getting up on stage on the truck and they said 'OutRage! has got a serious political message to say to everyone', and it went completely hushed. And I said 'You can never have enough shoes, handbags or gloves!'

JAMES KIERNEY

We had this cruising thing, where people put numbers on their backs. I had this number on my back, which I'd forgotten about, and I was on stage and my number was called out. I didn't realize, you had to go to the front, and this was someone I knew, a rent boy. I work with the homeless, and he was on the streets. I still see him, and I was quite embarrassed.

DICE

Since the summer before, we'd had a very hard time with the *Pink Paper*. This was the first time we'd had any positive press from the *Pink Paper*. Ben Summerskill was very appreciative of how cleverly we had been able to use the scene to disseminate leaflets and even collect some money, and it was OutRage! coming back to a position in community life. The procession involved a contingent from each of the bars and in subsequent years the whole thing has been appropriated to the letter by the bars. The year after, the first commercial version, there was a limp parade followed by a paid-entry event in St Anne's Park. Derek Jarman refused to pay to get into St Anne's Park.

STEVE COOK

With over 2000 people attending, the success of the Queer Carnival on 13 February 1993 was blighted by one major cloud. The previous December, after a series of financial irregularities over a number of years, the London Lesbian and Gay Centre had been declared bankrupt, and ceased to operate as a community centre. This left OutRage! with an uncertain future with regard to its office space. In the short term, the group effectively squatted in the Centre, refusing to be budged.

There were a series of bad appointments. There was no reason that the Centre could not be viable, but it was so badly, badly run. The bar was packed every night. Any pub could have made money on that.

LISA POWER

We were threatened with eviction from our office. We pretty much blockaded the office and had people there 24 hours a day. The first night, after this demand of us was made, we actually made sure there were people there overnight, to make sure they didn't break down the door. I was involved in negotiations with the chap who was the administrator of it all. He was in charge of issuing compensation as well. We felt we had a right to compensation, we'd had a tenancy there for quite a long time.

JOHN JACKSON

We ended up telling the receiver how to run their business. They had all sorts of weird ideas that they could slop us out, put their property in there. We managed to negotiate a pay-off from the receivers, which was very gratifying.

STEVE MAYES

We occupied the office on the last night. I remember turning up on the Saturday morning with a hammer and a crowbar, prepared to break into the building to occupy it.

STEVE COOK

Fortunately, the photographic association I was running was a hundred yards away round the corner, we had an empty floor. The place wasn't being used, it was a very convenient location for storing equipment, storing filing cabinets and all the rest of it. We managed to hold meetings there, we had a party, it was great because we didn't have to leave at a certain time. It went on until four in the morning. The office was essentially being run independently from people's homes. The filing cabinet, archive material, was there. There was no telephone, just storage.

STEVE MAYES

I moved us out of the LLGC to Steve Mayes's place. Things like plants had been abandoned, left there. I was saying let's take these, I thought it was really sad. People had been growing plants to make it a nice place and they got left behind… I drove over a nail and my tyre burst, [I remember] having to buy a new tyre and wondering whether I could claim from OutRage! for my new tyre.

LYNNE SUTCLIFFE

There was a lot of disruption and I don't think it did OutRage! any good, that move. There was less organization after that. In the Lesbian and Gay Centre, you'd get a lot of people who said 'Oh, I'm here now, I'll go down to the meeting and go take a look.' We'd get people walking in on the off-chance that something was happening. The people who stayed with OutRage! at that time became closer and worked a lot easier, but a lot of people stopped coming.

NICK CAVE

One of the places we met was in Red Lion Square, where we met twice I think in some hole in the wall, it just didn't work. We decided after a while that the Kirby Street meetings in my office weren't satisfactory because there was no furniture. So we sent out reconnaissance parties all over the place and they turned up the Central Club. Essentially, it had relatively good access, it was central, it was cheap.

STEVE MAYES

There were several venues for the Thursday meetings, including (for a couple of weeks) Covent Garden Community Centre, and the Central Club YMCA. Eventually, everyone realized that OutRage! needed to have an established office, as the contact point for the group during this time was David Allison's home number.

We'd been looking for an office and, just flicking through the *Evening Standard*, I found a number of locations. One in Dean Street, St Anne's Church Centre, we nearly got, but when they found out it was queers, they wouldn't let us in. A friend, who was a film editor, was using this office [in Peter Street, Soho], and had about three years of his lease left, and couldn't afford it, and was more than happy to pass the concern over to us. It was appallingly mishandled by his landlord who just had very, very bad legal advice. We, on the other hand, had quite good legal advice, and we managed to secure tenure of this place without a lease. We're in the fortunate position of not having any responsibilities whatsoever but having security of tenure. It's kind of grown-up stuff, getting a proper lease in a proper office in this area.

STEVE MAYES

We went in on a Saturday, ripped everything out and painted it, and the priorities were where to put the megaphones, the cupboard with all these outed people from history. There were all those icons from the lesbian and gay community that had come from the les/gay centre, little shrines or something. It was like moving house, in a completely random, distorted, dysfunctional family sort of way.

ROB KEMP

Stop in the name of love!

Throughout the move, OutRage! had continued with some of its ongoing actions, such as the Schools Initiative, zapping Harrow School in March and John Major's old school at Rutlish in South Wimbledon on 26 May.

It was a boys' school, they were all very supportive, we had no hassle down there at all. There was this bloke from the school magazine, I'm sure he was queer actually, but he took a great interest in it. The teachers were very friendly towards us.

DICE

Following the success of OutRage!'s involvement in the employment dispute with Royal Mail, other gay men and lesbians would approach OutRage! to support their cases against employers. One such case which OutRage! supported was that of Haringey Council worker David Morgan, zapping a meeting of the Council on 1 July.

I remember David Morgan and a Tory councillor coming along to a meeting at Steve Mayes's offices. David Morgan had been sacked from his job. Haringey Council was not enforcing its equal opportunities policy. He'd no problems with anyone there. We looked at the case and felt we should support it, and initially had some communication through the post with Haringey Council for a number of weeks. I remember David Morgan was very anxious that we get involved, and felt he had received no support from the gay community. He's been to Stonewall, got no support there, the queer Labour group, so he came to us. The action we decided to take was to invade the council offices.

We raided the council offices while the council was sitting. Somebody had got in in advance and was holding the door open for us. It was easier than expected. When we got into the meeting, the mayor was on his seat, we took over his microphone, which was still on. We tried to engage in conversation with some of the councillors. Most of the councillors got up and walked out. We stayed in the chamber for quite a while. We took photographs beside the councillors.

DICE

However, David Morgan's dismissal and appeal were not what was on the minds of the gay community during the summer of 1993. A series of gruesome murders led the Metropolitan Police to believe that a serial killer was targeting gay men and, with the Pride festival quickly on the horizon and threats allegedly from the killer to tabloid newspapers to kill a gay man a week, there was understandable anxiety within London's gay community. The murders had begun in March when a theatre director, Peter Walker, had been found in his flat with his wrists tied. In a later call to the *Sun* a man confessed that it had been his New Year's resolution to murder someone. On 30 May, librarian Chris Dunn was found dead wearing leather bondage gear, leading the police initially to treat his murder as an 'accident'. In early June, the bodies of Perry Bradley and Andrew Collier were found strangled in their flats, and on 15 June Emanuel Spiteri was found dead in his flat after his killer had attempted to set fire to it. That night, the police held a press conference to announce the fact they were dealing with a serial killer. The spectacle of SM-related murders, and the HIV-positive status of three of the men murdered, led to immediate media speculation about 'AIDS revenge murders', and various reports about the 'homosexual underworld'. In response to police suggestions that gay men shouldn't go home with strangers, Peter Tatchell suggested a more imaginative and appealing alternative; the police should encourage men to go home in groups, thereby advocating group sex.

Relationships between gay groups and the police became increasingly strained, with groups such as GALOP and OutRage! criticizing the police for not working with the gay community, and in particular for not appointing out gay police officers to the investigation. At Pride that year, the police distributed 400 posters and 10,000 leaflets amongst unprecedented media interest – with a serial killer on the loose, Pride became of interest for the mainstream press and media. At Pride, singer Sinitta made an emotional, if misplaced, appeal: 'If the murderer is out there – Stop! In The Name Of Love!' before launching into the song of the same name.

Eventually, the police did appoint an anonymous gay police officer to help with the enquiry on 6 July. The police admitted that the number of calls received rose. On 20 July, Colin Ireland was arrested and charged with five murders. The Colin Ireland murders were enough to persuade OutRage! that they were being used in a publicity exercise for the police.

We had a list of grievances as a result of the Colin Ireland case, but we also had a long-running dispute with the Policing Initiative, for example issues of police harassment of gay men cruising, their lack of specific banning of homophobic behaviours by members of the police force. It became the straw that broke the camel's back. When the Colin Ireland case came about, a lot of reports went out of their way to stress the close liaison that was occurring with the police, and the police on TV would mention 'Well, we have this wonderful thing called the Lesbian and Gay Policing Initiative', and it was that that made us feel we were not going to be used as a publicity exercise.

FERNANDO GUASCH

We realized it might take the police a while to shift from their old homophobic mind-set to a more gay-friendly one. We felt that the consultation with the gay community had basically become a PR exercise for the Metropolitan Police. We gave the police an ultimatum – either you start addressing these homophobic aspects of policing or we leave the group. We don't want to give you credibility when you're dragging your feet. Although some officers privately acknowledged the need to move faster and were concerned that gay disillusionment could undermine the whole process, they were in a minority and their objections were vetoed.

PETER TATCHELL

What we saw was queer groups becoming complicit with our oppressors. It gave the Met an opportunity to put their case. In fact, they were doing fuck all. It was the politics of appeasement, which is very common. It's an assimilationist tactic which allows the oppressor to walk away. OutRage! pulled out of the group, and it was seen at the time as a fiendish, awful thing to do, treacherous to the gay community. You can only achieve things by dissent and opposition, you can't do it by conciliation.

STEVE MAYES

We thought long and hard about the consequences of leaving, but knew that others of a more conservative nature would remain and could carry on the agenda. We just felt that we didn't want to waste our time with a body that wasn't doing any good. If others were prepared to do the hard slog, that was fine by us.

PETER TATCHELL

Although OutRage! left the Policing Initiative – the organization which they had, effectively, founded three years previously – they had inadvertently raised their own standing within the police force a month or so before. An unofficial, but recognized, friction between the Met and the Crown Prosecution Service resulted in the CPS being viewed as the bogies of the justice system by the police, unwilling and unable to convict following lengthy investigations. The CPS was also frequently the target of OutRage! criticisms concerning prosecutions against gay men. On 22 July, OutRage! zapped the CPS Head Office.

The Crown Prosecution Service was a real wheeze. We'd discovered that you could walk through a door, where you want, as you want, when you want. We talked about doing Scotland Yard. We checked out the security, realized we could have zapped them had we chosen to. The CPS was the next major thing. The CPS was being pernicious, very homophobic, in its application of law. They were very deliberately prosecuting queer things. They had just installed new security, which was basically a door, with a lock, and someone standing next to it with a badge on, a security guard. We just steamed in and filled the building, sent people to every floor, by lift, by stair, by whatever, filled the place with leaflets, telling everyone what was going on, why we were angry with them, and leave.

STEVE MAYES

We not only got into the building, we got into the Director of Public Prosecutions' office. We were actually standing there and one of the OutRage! members picked up the phone to make a press release and said 'We are in the DPP's office.'

NICK CAVE

We inadvertently zapped British Telecom. If you go into the building, there are two separate organizations. So, we still owe British Telecom a zap – they're allowed to be homophobic once, and they won't be zapped is the theory, because they've already been zapped. The police were called, and of course the police hate the CPS, so there was a really interesting situation where for the first time ever the police were very much on our side. I sold the photographs to the *Police Gazette*. They reported it salaciously, because they saw it as an opportunity to have a laugh at the CPS.

STEVE MAYES

Afterwards, Peter told us his source had overheard somebody speaking in the office, 'Thank God it was only OutRage!' So one of us wrote to the DPP and said 'What do you mean it was only OutRage! Dismiss us like that and we'll come back!' I believe they spent about £5 million on security after that.

NICK CAVE

The move from the LLGC had left OutRage! leaner and meaner than before. They were more confident in the zaps they could perform, and whom they could challenge. The abolition of the focus groups and the move away from the Centre had left them with a low public image, during which the group had to rely on each other for inspiration, direction and support. On the one hand, it made the group less accountable for the actions it took, while on the other hand it gave them much more licence for queer terrorism. On 26 August, OutRage! celebrated its third year of activism with a relaunch party, signalling an appetite for high-profile action once again.

NOTES

1 Michelangelo Signorile, *Queer In America: Sex, the Media and the Closets of Power* (Abacus, 1994), pp. 302–3. Geffen was also controversial because of his management of anti-gay comedian Andrew Dice Clay, whom he later dropped. Geffen's attitude changed markedly over the next couple of years, partly in response to a series of attacks on him by Signorile and other 'outers'. By the end of 1992, he was receiving an award from AIDS Project Los Angeles, coming out fully as a gay man and remarking that he'd 'come a long way'.

ELEVEN

Jeans, Genes, Stroppy Queens

In the summer of 1993, the old chestnut of 'What causes homosexuality?' had reared its head again, after the publication in a leading American publication, *Science*, of research into a 'gay gene'. Studying 40 pairs of homosexual brothers, a team from the US Government National Cancer Institute concluded that an X gene inherited from mothers may be responsible for making men gay. The research generated a debate on not only the cause of homosexuality, but what to do with information gained from such genetic research.

The research was shot down by the gay and lesbian media and politicos, not on the grounds that the 'evidence' was limited in scope and implication (which it was), but solely because it heretically suggested homosexuals were *made* rather than self-creating. Such a knee-jerk reaction to the issue of genetic markers for homosexuality is partly explained by an understandable fear/phantasy of a homophobic society tampering with genetics to block sexualities...The rejectionist stance of gay and lesbian communities on both sides of the Atlantic to the work of geneticists exemplifies the irrational attitudes that recur in gay and lesbian theory and politics; too often we find ourselves defending homosexualities from charges of intellectual hypocrisy and fraud.

CHRIS WOODS, *STATE OF THE QUEER NATION*[1]

The former Chief Rabbi, Lord Jakobovits, claimed that 'If we could by some form of genetic engineering eliminate these trends [homosexual tendencies], we should so long as it is done for a therapeutic purpose.' The current Chief Rabbi, Dr Jonathan Sacks, managed to distance himself somewhat from the comments, but Jakobovits's continued stance against homosexuality brought him into sharp conflict with OutRage!

We had a long debate on it. The first thing was 'My God, this is a real hornet's nest.'

FERNANDO GUASCH

We would approach a liberal synagogue with a view to debating with them what they thought of this, and how they would join us in lobbying Jakobovits to retract the statement. We did some research and found the Marble Arch synagogue.

STEVE MAYES

We had maybe two active Jewish members. [Jakobovits] echoed the kind of fascism that persecuted the Jews in the Second World War. It was causing a lot of angst and a lot of pain for Jewish gay people. He was basically legitimizing that point of view, which at that time was gaining ground, a lot of speculation about a gay gene.

JOHN JACKSON

It was already a controversial issue in the public domain. Liberal Jews and others had already been condemning this in the pages of the mainstream press as well as the *Jewish Chronicle*. We chose the Jewish New Year because it was the most high-profile event of the Jewish calendar and we chose a cosmopolitan synagogue right in the heart of London, where we thought a lot of different Jews would turn up on this day, to whom we could distribute this leaflet. In terms of tactics, it was one of the limpest things we could do.

STEVE COOK

[The leaflet had] some fairly provocative headings, a picture of Jakobovits, making a comparison of what Hitler was saying in 1933 and what Jakobovits was saying in '93. There were very few of us, we had two people posted either side of the door handing out leaflets, and on the other side of the street some people holding placards.

STEVE MAYES

We'd interrupted lots of church services before, but not synagogue services, and people found it very, very offensive that we had done that and the leaflet had images of the Holocaust on them which they couldn't believe we'd used. I don't know whether it would have had as much impact if we hadn't. I don't know if as many people would have talked about it if the images hadn't been quite as controversial. I thought it was right to do the zap.

LYNNE SUTCLIFFE

There was never a press release from OutRage! on this, it was not a public action. A synagogue attendant rang the police, the police told us, saying there were skinheads trying to break into the building.

FERNANDO GUASCH

There was an immediate panic and a dozen police cars, a few vans and dozens and dozens of policemen arrived. There was nothing happening! There was a very lively debate and we all went home.

STEVE MAYES

Chris Woods reported in *Capital Gay* 'OutRage! accused of anti-Semitism, a zap on a Jewish synagogue'. We were not even obstructing the pavement!'

FERNANDO GUASCH

A pernicious and absolutely ill-founded, factually inaccurate report, digging for anti-Semitic motivation for what we were doing. It snowballed, it forced a debate. The first few weeks in the gay press were very hostile to OutRage!, but as the arguments came back it moved. The debate got much more rational and it became evident that it was possible to criticize in a way which PC had prevented criticism in the past, to permit people to stand up and say 'I do not believe…'. If you're homophobic, you're homophobic. We were saying there was no defence for homophobia.

STEVE MAYES

The very analyses we made had already been spelled out by Jewish commentators in the pages of the *Jewish Chronicle*. I mentioned this [at a meeting with Hineinu, a Jewish gay group], that the very same arguments had been made by straight Jewish people. If you claim the argument becomes odious when used by gay people or gentiles then you presume that only straight Jewish people can criticize. The more we severed links with these groups, the more we could quite explicitly and consciously become the bad boys and girls who had nothing to lose.

FERNANDO GUASCH

OutRage! was labelled anti-Semitic for targeting a liberal Jewish synagogue because of the actions of a right-wing Jewish man. Undeterred by the criticisms made of them, OutRage! also supported a Welsh gay direct action group, Dicclon, which demonstrated against Jakobovits when he received an award from the University of Wales in Cardiff on 30 November.

The sorry saga of the Benetton Nine

Benetton, the target of ACT UP and OutRage! fury the year before in 1992 over their AIDS imagery in adverts, had begun an even more controversial advertising campaign earlier in 1993, involving the phrase 'H.I.V. POSITIVE' being tattooed onto three parts of a naked figure. Claiming they had the support of the London Lighthouse and the Terrence Higgins Trust, some adverts in the press also contained the contact number for the National AIDS Helpline. The Terrence Higgins Trust and London Lighthouse both denied endorsing the campaign, claiming that only after the images had been sent to a number of magazines were they consulted, at which point they had suggested including the National AIDS Helpline number after being shocked at the images used.

I was the only one in the group who didn't have a problem with this. I made a speech saying I thought it was OK, and I remember suddenly feeling on the outside, somehow I'd said the wrong thing. Fernando said 'Traitor, traitor' and although it was a joke, there was a sense I had been a traitor, because I'd spoken out.

GRAHAM KNIGHT

We had spent the previous month phoning Benetton. They are so adept at twisting every piece of criticism, and wearing it like a hat. When we discovered Luciano Benetton published complaint letters in some nice bound edition, we realized we did not want to give them anything that was going to give them substance. We did not want any press at all. We thought the building was going to be their headquarters and the impact would be felt in Italy half an hour later. I was a bit worried because a woman had turned up, Helen, who had never done an action of this type, and she was quite nervous.

FERNANDO GUASCH

The Benetton Nine were myself, Ben Croll, Martin Corbett, Billy Stuart, David Swinburne, Chris Tyler, Fernando, Helen from ACT UP and Dice. It was this building in a residential area in Fulham, so it was difficult for a gang of people to creep up on the building without being seen. The plan was, Billy would go slightly ahead. They let him in, he picked up some brochures and then when he was coming out he dropped the brochures on the floor, so he'd have this excuse to keep the door open while he picked up his papers.

STEVE COOK

One of the reasons we knew we had been tapped was because it was put together, literally, in 48 hours. We had only used the phone twice from the OutRage! office the night before, so we were surprised to see the police when we turned up.

FERNANDO GUASCH

I was the link between Billy and the gang of people. At the time Billy was in the building, the Security Guard came out and started chatting to the policeman stood outside. The policeman came across the road to me and said something like 'Hello'. He said 'Are you here for the demo?' and I said 'What demo? I'm here waiting for a bus.' He just went, 'Oh, OK,' and crossed back over. I saw Billy coming out. I waved to the group at the same time as I was crossing the road and decided the only thing I could do was engage the policeman in conversation as the group was creeping up from behind, and it worked like a dream. The policeman turned to me as I was crossing the road, so he had his back to the protesters and I said 'What demo's this, then?' He said, 'Oh well, you don't need to know if you're not involved.' I said 'Well it's not going to be a very big demo, there's nobody here!' By that time, most people had crept in literally behind his back. The Security Guard, who'd also been talking to me, saw them out of the corner of his eye. They just managed to catch Ben Croll, the last person creeping in behind their backs.

STEVE COOK

Most of us overshot, past the door, into the car park. The security was such that we were able to retrace our steps! We were all expecting long corridors, a lot of space to run amok with foghorns. However, we were faced with a very narrow building with two rooms on each level, so we had no room to move. We went to the top floor and hung placards from the windows.

FERNANDO GUASCH

There were largely middle-aged women employees there, and we went round saying to them 'Don't be alarmed, it's just a protest, nothing's going to happen', and that came out in court with some of the more honest witnesses.

STEVE COOK

We heard the sirens, I could see them from the window, two if not three vans. We said 'We're leaving now, we're not doing anything.' They were just grabbing people and throwing them down the stairs. I was flung down.

FERNANDO GUASCH

They weren't just police, they were SRG [Special Response Group], with almost body armour, and they piled in. They broke the front door down, real drama queens, rushed all the way up the staircase and grabbed everyone. The staircase was like your mother's staircase, really narrow.

STEVE COOK

Normally, they ask us to leave the building, it's as simple as that. We weren't asked, we were simply attacked. They went for me because I was taking photographs. I'd taken photographs of some of the police assaulting some of the demonstrators. They got us outside, roughed us up, I was thrown against a wall. They took the camera off me, put cuffs on, really, really tight.

DICE

The police piled the protesters into vans, and took them to the station where they were kept for several hours. Initially, the charge was going to be breaking and entering, but most of the group were eventually charged with Section 4 of the relatively new Public Order Act, with behaviour likely to cause someone to fear violence. Two of the protesters, Ben Croll and Martin Corbett, were charged with assaulting the police. When the case came to court, OutRage! were able to furnish a first-class defence team in gay lawyer Angus Hamilton, Sue Green and barrister Mark Guthrie who had often offered their services to groups like OutRage! and ACT UP on previous occasions.

Part of the terms of my bail was that I wasn't allowed near a Benetton store. I remember taking great pride in going to Benetton stores in Glasgow, and London as well.

DICE

There was a five-day trial, during which we heard the police one after another perjuring themselves and contradicting themselves. [The solicitors] were brilliant, they just pissed on all the evidence. They pissed on the CPS [Crown Prosecution Service] who were pathetic, but we only got off in the end because of the incompetence of the CPS guy, who failed to ask the one question he needed to ask the Benetton witnesses, which was 'Did you at any time fear violence might be done to you?' If they'd have said yes to that, we'd have gone down and we could have got three months. It was quite an enjoyable trial. There was a lot of drama, we were all very good in the dock, and the magistrate was lovely, she was an eccentric.

STEVE COOK

They were saying things outrageous – and this was one of the top police officers who swore on the bible – that we were holding placards on wooden sticks and we were using these wooden sticks as weapons against the police. We had photographs – we had A2 pieces of paper!

FERNANDO GUASCH

There was a police line about what had happened on the day. They said I'd said something like 'Let's get these police bastards.' Presumably, they said that because I was the photographer and they'd damaged the camera and the film, so most of the photos wouldn't develop, which was very 'convenient'. The magistrate seemed to recognize that the police were lying. We got a lot of support from the community. We were dubbed 'The Benetton Nine'. I never felt we were going to get convicted. We never really did anything wrong. Section 4 was very new at the time, it needed to be qualified in court.

DICE

Helen, because it was her first action, spoke very movingly about how she had become involved because she'd nursed a close friend up until the point of his death. The magistrate was clearly impressed by the personal involvement of people. In the trial, it became clear that we'd been bugged in some way or other. [Our solicitor] had this computer aided dispatch [printout] and she said 'What do the letters "SB" stand for?' Apparently, there had been some kind of notification in the local police station at 6.45 in the morning that OutRage! would be descending on the building. This was hours before we were anywhere near the area. On Sue Green asking 'What does "SB" stand for?' he said 'Well, in my experience it stands for Special Branch.'

FERNANDO GUASCH

We had some brilliant character witnesses, a Professor of Chinese at Oxford, with whom the magistrate debated the niceties of Chinese calligraphy. My boyfriend's father, who's a retired Presbyterian minister, came as my character witness and stood there in his dog collar with a disarming Geordie accent, saying 'I would have been proud if my daughter had brought home Steve as a prospective husband, but as it is, he makes a great companion for my son.' [The Magistrate] obviously thought we were misguided but honourable people. We got off.

STEVE COOK

I wanted them to get off, but what got them off is the fact that we've got very good lawyers whereas a lot of people won't have and, secondly, we've got this group of very well educated people who've got these impressive qualifications that are working in their favour.

LYNNE SUTCLIFFE

The following year, in June 1994, Benetton offered funding to the organizers of the 'Quilts of Love' open-air exhibition of panels from the AIDS memorial quilt in Hyde Park. OutRage! warned the Edinburgh Names Project that Benetton would be troublesome funders. Benetton and the organizers of Quilts Of Love agreed that Benetton would produce 25,000 commemorative programmes at a cost of £26,000, as long as the event organizers had total editorial control over the content. Benetton also then went on to produce 25,000 'resource guides' to be inserted into the programmes, which turned out not only to be inaccurate, but also reproduced their controversial tattoo advert. Volunteers had to stay up late into the night to stamp over a Benetton logo on the inside front cover of the programme, as it gave the impression that Benetton had funded the entire event. On the day of the exhibition, Steve and Fernando followed Benetton's PR Manager, Marysia Woroniecka, around the site, challenging her at every opportunity.

I was just livid, I wanted blood. The organizers, who could not be seen to be supporting us, kept chasing us the whole day, saying 'You're doing the work of God… she's in the PR tent.' I remember going up to her in the PR tent, she didn't know who I was. I introduced myself and began, in front of everyone, showing her the programme and calling her a ghoul and a carrion eater who was feeding on the corpses of my friends.

FERNANDO GUASCH

She was trying to chuck us out, saying 'They're not press, they're not press.' So Edward King came along and said 'I'm press, I write for the *Pink Paper*'. He tackled her because this programme had a resource guide which was full of inaccuracies.

STEVE COOK

Queerying the Minister

In November, even though it had recently left the London Policing Initiative, OutRage! was still exerting pressure on the Met. Gay men at cruising grounds were still being regularly harassed by police, and on 12 November, Peter Tatchell went to deliver a letter on behalf of OutRage! to New Scotland Yard.

While there, he noticed an unusually high level of activity and was told that the Prime Minister was due to arrive at any moment.

I went into the nearby building society and made enquiries about opening an account and pretended to fill in a form, all the time discreetly looking out for the arrival of the Prime Minister's car. As soon as it came into view, I waited until he got out of the car and just at the moment when he was being greeted by the Commissioner I began running full pelt across the forecourt, darting between two policemen and somehow hurtling a three foot high barrier. I managed to get within ten feet before I was tackled to the ground by four uniformed officers and Special Branch. By this time, the Prime Minister and the Commissioner were giving a joint press conference just a few feet away. I shouted out 'Prime Minister – why do you support anti-gay discrimination? Why won't you vote for an equal age of consent for gay men?' The police kept trying to put their hands across my mouth but I kept yanking away and repeating the questions. Evidently it was being picked up on all the television coverage, and the Prime Minister kept turning round and looking at me as if to say to the police 'Why can't you shut the fucker up?'

PETER TATCHELL

Tatchell's shouting prevented the press conference from being held, and after the Prime Minster and the Chief Commissioner had gone inside Scotland Yard, Peter was taken off and given a sharp dressing down by the police, but not arrested. Rather surprised that he had got off so lightly, Peter went to unlock his bike and return to the OutRage! office.

All of a sudden I noticed from out of the corner of my eye that Major and [Commissioner] Condon had come outside again and were resuming the press conference. I thought, 'They're not going to get away with this', so I pedalled full pelt and drove straight at them. I got within eight or ten feet before I was felled by the police. Again I shouted out 'Why won't you support homosexual equality' and again, the press conference had to be abandoned, this time for good. I was held for a while before an officer came over and said 'They're not coming out again, so you can let him go.'

PETER TATCHELL

By now, the almost traditional OutRage! zap on the State Opening of Parliament was also looming, with OutRage! planning again to protest, which they did on 18 November.

We told the police we'd be demonstrating and duly turned up with our banners and placards. We challenged them months in advance to find a reason to stop us, every one we were able to rebut. On the day, they had no reason to stop us, they simply arrested us because they didn't like it, which to my mind was profoundly important. It exposed the role of the police, it just stripped them naked. It's a lesson I carry to this day. If there's an example of how the State operates, that was it in a nutshell.

STEVE MAYES

Yet it wasn't all ministerial and parliamentary zaps in the latter part of 1993. Towards the end of the year, two major actions exhibited the extent of OutRage!'s intervention in 'straight' society, claiming (and promoting) queer space. To celebrate World AIDS Day the previous year, OutRage! had zapped the offices of Durex protesting at their refusal to promote extra-strong condoms for anal intercourse, or amongst the gay community.

On World AIDS Day 1993, OutRage! followed up on some of their schools actions. Targeting the Sixth Form College of Christ the King in Lewisham, a Catholic school, OutRage! developed a safer-sex pack to distribute amongst the children during a lunch break. Using their contact with the Terrence Higgins Trust, they managed to get a range of leaflets, condoms and lubricant sachets to give away.

Acknowledging that it had been a turbulent year, and that OutRage! had managed to survive a number of difficult patches throughout 1992 and 1993, the group also organized a fun queer outing. Harking back to the WIG assault on Oxford Street, OutRage! arranged a queer glamorous assault on heterosexual Saturday shoppers on 18 December, followed by a party at Kirby Street in the evening.

I manifested briefly as a nun, but it's something I wasn't very good at. I was Sister Sporran. I thought it was portraying a stereotypical image of queers as happy, passive funny people who dressed up strange. We handed out cards.

DICE

Peter dressed up as Father Christmas. He put chains round his neck and big placards saying 'Father Christmas says...' He'd been drunk the night before, mind you. I found that out. He'd been to a Stonewall party.

BETH LANE

Fernando wore a black cocktail dress and a huge long black curly wig, stilettos and a machine gun. Peter just wore his normal outfit with a Father Christmas hat on top, really. Peter never liked dressing up.

LYNNE SUTCLIFFE

The party at Kirby Street was a chance for the group to socialize, after a hard day's drag. Even as the celebrations were going on, everyone in the group was aware that 1994 had a major challenge ahead for them; the debate about an equal age of consent was gathering momentum, with a bill likely to go through Parliament in the early part of the New Year. Having campaigned for an equal age of consent for as long as it had been in existence, the issue was very close to their hearts. For the first time since 1967, there was serious talk about an equal age of consent for gay men.

NOTE

1   Chris Woods, *State of the Queer Nation: A Critique of Gay and Lesbian Politics in 1990s Britain* (Cassell, 1995), p. 4.

TWELVE

The Riot That Nearly Was

The Stonewall Group had already been challenging the age of consent laws through the European Courts, after identifying a couple, Hugo Greenhalgh and Will Parry, who had 'confessed' to under-age sex. The police had decided not to prosecute the pair in September 1993, and preparations were well underway to take the British government to court in Europe by the time that Edwina Currie made an amendment to the Criminal Justice Bill in 1994. Tory MP Currie proposed an equal age of consent at 16, in what other members of her party privately referred to as 'The Buggers' Charter'.

OutRage! was also marshalling resources to put pressure on MPs to vote for an equal age of consent at 16. Concerned that much of the campaigning work was taking place behind closed doors, OutRage! decided it would organize a vigil outside the Houses of Parliament when the debate and vote were due to take place on 21 February. Earlier that month, Stonewall had a major fundraising show, Equality Now, to bring celebrities and famous supporters of an equal age of consent on board. In their zealousness to woo the famous and the mainstream media, they largely ignored the gay press, bringing them under fire that not only were they unelected, but arrogant and out of tune with lesbians and gay men on the street.

As the date for the House of Commons vote drew close, it also became clear that another amendment, which would be of favour to many in the Conservative Party, would be put forward. Sir Anthony Durant's amendment called for an age of consent for gay men set at the 'compromise' age of 18 – surely a compromise which could satisfy no one.

Joining forces with Stonewall, OutRage! advertised and organized for a mass peaceful presence outside Parliament as the debate went on – a visible reminder that the gay community was no longer invisible, and that the laws debated in the chambers would affect the lives of real people in an everyday sense. The vigil was given immediate poignancy in early February when one of OutRage!'s loudest supporters, film-maker Derek Jarman, died from HIV-related illness. It is said that his last words were that he wanted the world to be full of fluffy pink bunnies. The vigil became not only a mass demonstration, but a memorial to the uncompromising life of Derek Jarman as activist and artist.

On a cold and bitter night, almost 5000 lesbians, gay men and their supporters gathered in Parliament Square for the result of the vote. Despite the large numbers, the crowd was peaceful and good-hearted, singing the Sisters of Perpetual Indulgence anthem 'Amazing Pride' and the gay classic 'Somewhere Over the Rainbow' before observing a minute's silence in memory of Derek Jarman.

There were massive tensions between Stonewall and everyone else, because they were as usual pissing on everyone else. The candle lit vigil was definitely ours, although they came on board. I remember someone saying, 'Well, what if we lose?' Somebody said, 'Well, there'll be a riot, won't there?' I think we partly wanted it to happen. We turned up quite early. It was bitterly cold. Gradually, more and more and more people came. It was an extraordinary evening, looking down the road, this sea of people, a sea of candles. It seemed like there were many, many thousands, the lights up and down. The mood was optimistic. We genuinely thought we'd win.

ROB KEMP

It was pure chance that I was down in London for the age of consent vote. I met this bloke from Liverpool who I'd copped off with, and he lived in London. So I came down that weekend to stay with him, for a shag basically. He said there was this demonstration, and I talked to him about OutRage! and couldn't find out much. I found myself outside the House of Commons with thousands of others, very angry queers screaming and chanting. It was one of the most amazing nights of my life, it was just fantastic.

STUART COLLEY

I was in the distinguished strangers' gallery, courtesy of Christopher Spence. I was the person who stood up at the end and said 'Thanks for nothing', to which some sarcastic Tory bastard said 'You're welcome.' I'd just gone to work for Christopher Spence [Director of London Lighthouse], and I thought 'Oh my god. He's never going to speak to me again.' He thought it was quite funny, actually. He was quite pleased somebody had done it. There were all these gay men around me from radical groups, most of them were crying. I remember running to get outside. I rang a friend who'd asked me to ring her with the result. Poor

Christopher Spence emerged into the chanting mob who had heard the result and were really pissed off. He looked like a Tory MP, poor man, and they were ready to tear his liver out. I was stood on the steps inciting the crowd.

LISA POWER

It came out that we had lost, and everyone I knew wept. We'd done so much, we'd come so far, and we'd so clearly won the argument. We really should have won. Stonewall's initial response was, 'We're halfway there.' We were like 'Fuck bollocks we're halfway there. We've got nothing, we've got less than nothing.'

ROB KEMP

I remember people from Stonewall trying to speak to the crowd, and I was thinking 'You're mad, get out. This is no time to try and make people behave reasonably. They're fucking angry and they've got every right to be. This is not the time for Stonewall.' Edwina Currie, who's an excitable person at the best of times, complained that there was a rabble outside who were causing trouble. People were terribly well behaved. Ian McKellen went outside and looked at the crowd and said 'No, they're all being really well behaved.'

LISA POWER

I had this OutRage! banner that I'd managed to purloin off someone, 'Stroppy Queens Demand 16' which I was passing down Whitehall. Angela Mason came out, I think that's what really kicked it off. When Angela Mason announced that it was 18, and that this was a victory, nobody there was having it at all.

STUART COLLEY

I remember one of the Sisters (out of habit) talking to the crowd. The police moved in and removed the Sister, dragged him inside the Palace of Westminster. A friend from OutRage! tried to pull the Sister back, to stop the police arresting him, so he immediately got pulled in. I attended in a dog collar. As soon as my two friends had been pulled into the Palace of Westminster, I ran over and started banging on the doors, obviously couldn't do anything, but being a drama queen… at this point the police grabbed me, but the crowds had surged forward and grabbed me back. A court case ensued!

NICK CAVE

I thought OutRage! were a load of wankers, because of the press coverage. I only saw OutRage! in the straight press. Myself and a lot of other people got fired up and annoyed and angry, and also thrilled. Suddenly, you could be powerful. I think I turned a corner. You were within five minutes of getting through the door. It was that feeling of 5000 stroppy queens and you really could do things.

PHIL JONES

[I remember] falling over and getting trodden on and thinking 'I'm going to get trampled to death', not being able to get up, and Shaun, who's not particularly big, leaning in and pulling me up. I'd come straight from school and I was wearing a skirt and someone trod on my skirt, my skirt ripped and the button came off my shoe. I was thinking, 'There's my teacher's outfit gone to pot.'

LYNNE SUTCLIFFE

There was a guy climbing up the statute, with a pink flag which we'd taken along. The *Mail* or something the next day said, 'Protestors waved the red flag.' The guy with the flag managed to get away in the crowd. It just became a screaming mob, there was so much emotion there.

ROB KEMP

I remember walking back to Whitehall, stopping the traffic in Trafalgar Square, sitting in front of a No. 38 bus at Cambridge Circus, not allowing this bus to get to Shaftesbury Avenue and thinking 'You're going to have to run me over, because I'm so pissed off.' I was really, really angry.

ALAN JARMAN

It was the most single-minded riot I've ever seen, because if you map it out, it was actually making a bee-line for Jeremy Joseph's disco, and it stopped along the way – it stopped at 10 Downing Street, it stopped at Trafalgar Square, and it stopped at Cambridge Circus. I remember Martin Corbett shouting 'Let's take Old Compton Street' and somebody else saying, 'I think we've already got it!'

LISA POWER

We went past Waterstone's on Charing Cross Road, and put candles in front of the store [which had a Derek Jarman display], which was a really peaceful thing to do, considering we were all so angry.

ALAN JARMAN

One of the speakers to address the crowd after the vote had been announced, and the only one to be enthusiastically received, Peter Tatchell promised that the campaign for an equal age of consent would continue. The opportunity for direct action on the issue came about sooner than expected.

On the night of the age of consent vote someone anonymously came up to me and said 'You might be interested to know the Prime Minister is going to be opening a new unit at King's College Hospital in South London in two day's time.' He gave me a map of the hospital together with times of the Prime Minister's arrival and departure. I discussed this informally with other OutRage! members after the age of consent riot and we held an emergency meeting with a view to challenging John Major face to face.

PETER TATCHELL

That there should be an action against the Prime Minister was not in doubt – the only real thing to ascertain was how. There was a high level of security in London anyway, as the IRA had a bombing campaign underway, and OutRage! was only too aware that any of its direct action zaps could easily be misinterpreted as terrorist assassination attempts. With only five members available at such short notice, it was decided to attempt to disrupt the opening ceremony as the Prime Minister unveiled the new unit. Splitting into two groups on arrival, OutRage! tried to find an access point but, with the high level of security around, was unable to locate a suitable zap point. It decided to try a different tack – zapping John Major's cavalcade as it left the hospital.

We stood at a bus stop at Denmark Hill ostensibly reading newspapers. When John Major's motorcade came out of the hospital, we allowed the outriders and the first police car to pass and then ran out into the middle of the road and held our placards up, 'Consent At 16'. We'd emphasized the importance of holding the placards with both hands clearly above our heads to show we didn't have guns. The Prime Minister's car swerved sharply across the other side of the road, into the incoming lane. John Major's car came within five or six feet of me. I could see his face clearly in the window, it was a look of shock and horror and then he dived down on his seat with his hands clasped behind his head, which is presumably an anti-terrorist manoeuvre. We like to boast that OutRage! is the group that forced John Major to bend over for gay men.

PETER TATCHELL

OutRage! also began organizing for a March for Equality. On 14 March, nearly 2000 protesters gathered to break the Sessional Orders again and protest against Parliament, despite a massive police turn-out which included at least 35 vans and officers on horseback. The police formed a cordon across the lower part of the Haymarket as protesters marched down it. The group lay down in the road and chanted.

Steve Cook sidled up to me and went 'Are you still as "anti-Trot" as you've always been?' and I went 'Yes, of course, Steve', and he went 'Keep an eye on the SWP!' We'd said no sticks or any possible weapons were to be taken on the demonstration and the SWP had brought their placards on sticks. I said to Steve 'Find me someone tall, preferably with a working-class accent, in case they start on me.' Nick de Marco and LGCARF were there. When people were sat down in the Haymarket we identified a tiny group that we'd had our eyes on and they had a loudhailer. When they started saying 'We got to march on Parliament! Smash the pigs' I'd step in. By that time, my minder was Aamir and he went for them. I think Martin Corbett had to pull him off. Eventually we had to confiscate their loudhailer because they were inciting a riot! It cost the Metropolitan Police a million pounds in overtime. As you got into Westminster, they were everywhere!

MARTIN MAYNARD

We were outside Downing Street chanting. There were particular allegations about two Cabinet Ministers. John Major apparently had got back into Downing Street and I was subsequently told by people close enough to know that he was dying to come to the window to hear the chants, but he couldn't, so someone in his office rang up someone the next day and said 'Do you know anyone who was out there last night, because we'd like to know what they were chanting?' That person rang me, and I said 'Oh, they were chanting this about Lilley and Portillo', and he relayed it back to John Major's office. Given his attitude to Lilley and Portillo, I suspect he quite enjoyed it.

LISA POWER

The police kept making barriers across the road. I saw Peter Tatchell look to move us on, to move forward. As I moved forward, the two coppers in front of me literally moved together, they pushed me. I thought, 'Well if you're pushing me around...' so I gave them a push. The next thing, I remember Rob Kemp, the legal observer, standing right by me, watching. I lay down in the road, the coppers picked me up and carried me. I remember saying 'I'll walk, I'll walk', and Rob Kemp saying 'Are they hurting you?' I said 'Yes, they're hurting my arm.' The next thing I can remember was the doors of a van being opened and me being thrown in. I was charged with obstructing the police in the course of their duty and obstructing the public highway. I pleaded not guilty. They advised me to accept a caution, so I accepted a caution.

KEVIN

A more light-hearted stunt – although technically more serious in that it was a form of treason – was OutRage!'s invitation to Denmark to invade and impose their more liberal laws on homosexuality. In April, OutRage! demonstrated outside the Danish embassy in London calling for it to invade.

Peter burned the Union Jack, raising the new flag, which was a mixture of the Danish flag and the Union Jack. It was treason, because we were inviting another country to invade. It's still a hanging offence. None of us were hanged.

DICE

The bizarrest thing I ever did was calling for Denmark to invade. And then we stood there, and we didn't really know what to do. We had a drumming thing, a presentation. When we finished, we felt 'What have we done?' I'll never forget how stupid I felt at the end of it.

GRAHAM KNIGHT

More controversially, OutRage! targeted Labour, for their role in allowing the age of consent to be fixed at 18. Thirty-five Labour MPs – including Ann Taylor, David Blunkett, Stuart Bell, Joe Ashton, Dale Campbell-Savours, Bob Cryer, Stan Orme and Denzil Davies – voted against an equal age of consent, despite Labour having a policy for 'equality'. For months, rumours of an OutRage! zap on Labour had been circulating, but action had been postponed after gay Labour activists promised OutRage! that major policy promises would be forthcoming from the new Labour Party Leader, John Smith. With such promises not coming forth, OutRage! planned a zap for April at the Party's National Executive Meeting.

Fernando contacted them claiming to be from a Catalonian socialist group, coming along to ask some questions.

DICE

John Jackson was my son' and I had to pretend that I'd come down to London and my membership hadn't arrived – I had to find a false address quickly – and they had to go and hunt for it. Of course, they couldn't find it so they were looking for ages. We kept getting obstreperous and saying 'What on earth is going on? It must be there!' Then someone else came in and said he had a meeting. He had all these papers and kept dropping them, and everybody else went up at that point. John Jackson and I left smartly and stood outside with the placards.

BETH LANE

Beth was throwing a wobbly, saying 'You've lost my membership card, and I need another one soon because I want to get involved in the upcoming election.' They were making a great kerfuffle at the desk. We walked right past security, we had a map of the building, we rushed upstairs and we just stormed it.

FERNANDO GUASCH

The first person we saw when we walked in was Tony Blair, who was not sat at the table for some reason, but with the onlookers at the side. We went straight through, round the backs of people at the table. I remember standing behind Gordon Brown, who said 'Hi'.

STEVE COOK

We threw feathers. I stood behind David Blunkett and put my hand on his shoulders and said 'Don't be alarmed, this is a peaceful demonstration.' Gordon Brown stood up and said 'Who put you up to this?' I said 'No one put us up to this.' He said 'Who are you?' I said 'We're OutRage!'

DICE

They were absolutely convinced it was a Tory Party or Liberal Party put-up, and they would not believe it was OutRage! It was like some absurd political farce. I had the camera, so I had to go to the side of Blunkett and Smith so I could take photographs whereas everybody else aimed to go behind them and hold placards above their heads and throw white feathers and rubber chickens. They were very quick to launch on us, particularly me because I had the camera. They were totally afraid of any bad publicity, so they were really heavy. I managed to hold onto the camera, I think I put it down my trousers.

STEVE COOK

I was thrown down the stairs. I managed to grab on to the banister, regain my posture. They were being quite violent towards us. They didn't want the police to throw us out, so they did it themselves.

DICE

We put posters all over the front door. They'd locked the front door, and we did a rendition of 'The Pink Flag' and then the main effort was to try and get the film developed, to see if there was a good enough photo of John Smith. We had some photos, as evidence of what we'd done.

STEVE COOK

They issued a statement denying it [had taken place]. Subsequently, John Smith died, and they said it was because of us!

DICE

The zap on the Labour Party Executive was mirrored the same month by an OutRage! Merseyside zap on MP Bob Parry. The Merseyside demo was part of a pay-off to OutRage! for giving them a broken fax machine, which OutRage! Merseyside had managed to mend.

Continuing with high-profile public marches and actions on the theme of the age of consent, OutRage! organized an event which repeated the 1992 Teenage Turn-In, emphasizing the fact that 17-year-old men – who, if heterosexual, would be legally able to have sex – would still be prosecuted under the changed law. Despite attempts by OutRage! to obtain undertakings from the government and from the police that such prosecutions would not be in the public interest, the likelihood remained that prosecutions and imprisonments would happen. The Teenage Turn-In took place at Charing Cross Police Station on 7 May.

I remember it was on the radio that morning and one 17-year-old turned up because he'd been doing his homework and suddenly decided to come down. The Zimbabwe Embassy was just outside the police station and the statues have got bits of their bodies lopped off – they've got heads, they're naked, and it was considered indecent. It wasn't considered so indecent if they didn't have heads, because then they're not like real people. I gave a speech saying the laws about decency, that made people chop heads off statues, are still the same laws that are getting people now for having sex under-age.

LYNNE SUTCLIFFE

When I was still 16 I went on the Teenage Turn-In outside Charing Cross Police Station. I heard about that because I saw a poster for it on a toilet door at the Angel Bar in Islington. I hadn't been there on the 1st February, and I really wanted to, I was at home, with the radio, crying my eyes out, because I was still in the closet to my parents. I came out precisely because of the vote, I thought I just couldn't keep it in anymore. I went along to the Turn-In. I was immediately part of the action, I was right at the front. I saw myself on *London Tonight*. Afterwards we were all invited for a drink at Halfway to Heaven, but for some stupid reason, I was too shy to go. Brave enough to go on the action, but too shy to go for a drink!

MARINA CRONIN

The birth of the Lesbian Avengers

The age of consent campaign had focused almost exclusively on gay men, as this was where the most obvious discrimination lay. For some, however, it pointed up the historical difficulty of women's involvement within OutRage!

I enjoyed working with the men in OutRage! By this stage, none of the old women were left, there was just me and Beth. I thought the age of consent campaign had excluded a lot of women, because it wasn't seen as an issue that affected women. We did this questionnaire, which was deliberately controversial. 'Do you think it would better to make us less invisible in the eyes of the law so we can be legally discriminated against or are there other issues that you would like to work around more?' It listed some issues, and then had a space for others. We gave them out at Pride, we put them in 2000 issues of *Diva*. I got hundreds and hundreds back and there was a box [to tick] saying if you want to receive more information from OutRage! and not many people did. The test for me was whether there were women out there who wanted to do anything at this point or not. I thought it's not going to be via OutRage!, I have to face up to that really, so let's try a different strategy.

LYNNE SUTCLIFFE

Lynne met up with fellow activist Roz Hopkins, and then met some activists from a group which had recently started in America. The Lesbian Avengers was founded in June 1993 by six lesbian activists who wanted a direct action group to fight for lesbian survival and visibility. Roz and Lynn began to discuss the feasibility of starting up a similar group in Britain and produced a leaflet setting up an initial meeting on 26 August, distributing 300 leaflets around the bars.

Seventy women turned up to a very small room that we'd booked in the Central Club with a donation from OutRage! We planned to show a video of the American Avengers and we'd got a portable TV. I thought there are so many women here, I've got to do something. It's obvious that they want their own group and they want to work with women. The energy in that room that night was fantastic, I was almost drunk with it. I'd spent months with one or two women coming to OutRage! It was obvious the time was right, it wasn't right the year before, it was now. I think it was partly a backlash against the lesbian chic thing and it was time for real lesbians to take lesbianism back, an agenda that was real for them.

LYNNE SUTCLIFFE

The success of the first meeting led to further meetings, and the setting up of Lesbian Avengers in the UK. The Avengers started their own zaps by protesting next to Queen Victoria's statue at Buckingham Palace on 26 August – the woman alleged to have encouraged lesbian invisibility.

I didn't want to leave OutRage! at first. I can remember people saying to me, 'You mustn't leave OutRage! because you're one of the few women that we've got' and me saying 'I can do both', Steve Mayes saying 'You can't say that to her, she's got to do what she thinks is right. I don't think she's going to have the time and energy to do both. There's something happening that we can't deny or stop.' I had to stop at that point and think 'There are no longer 70 or 60 or 50 or even 40 people involved in OutRage! now and it's time to reassess.' It's very hard to let go of something that has been so powerful. OutRage! and Avengers did some good work together.

LYNNE SUTCLIFFE

OutRage! – the tour

The age of consent campaigns highlighted differences between the tactics and aims of OutRage! and Stonewall. Friction between the two groups became increasingly apparent and at one point the Stonewall Chair announced her 'personal displeasure' at the OutRage! zap on the Labour Party. Although, in the early days, OutRage! and Stonewall had recognized that they worked differently, they had been able to work together and often cooperated in organizing actions and press campaigns. By 1994, there was a sharp contrast in style and message.

[In 1990] Shane became my gardener, which caused a certain amount of gyp in Stonewall, because we used to have the Stonewall board meeting while he was hauling the garden rubbish in and out. Michael Cashman, who quite fancied him, said 'That man in your house is from OutRage!, he could have been listening to anything!' Shane and I used to let each other know what our organizations were doing, so there was a little link. There was some public posturing, but nothing very serious. It was all fairly pragmatic. Shane and I trusted each other. There was nobody left at OutRage! who trusted Stonewall and so it got very bitter.

LISA POWER

The influence on Stonewall I think was the Spring '93 March on Washington, where they all went over, saw what an incredible job the

National Task Force had done and started to think 'we too could control the lesbian/gay political agenda and be a real in-your-face public pom-pom-waving organization.' From that point onwards, they started to change dramatically and I think that had a dramatic effect on how they were seen by OutRage! I thought Parliament was not important to people's lives so much as what the community thought of itself. An era had dawned when lesbians and gay men were in the mainstream, we can get our rights through Parliament, everything will be jolly, we can carry on partying. I saw Stonewall as representing all the worst features that had come to the fore of the lesbian and gay community over the years since 1992 – the rate of commercialism, the decline of activism.

STEVE COOK

We thought we'd get involved in Pride. By then, we were already involved in the Pride March Committee. We attended quite a few of those meetings without Stonewall being there at all. We made banners, it was supposed to be every area that might affect lesbians and gays. It was a highly elaborate display. Each banner would have 'Housing Rights', whatever, followed by lollipop signs, each point of law.

FERNANDO GUASCH

Through their Press Officer Roger Goode, they were issuing press releases on Pride Trust headed paper, saying that this year – thanks to Stonewall – there were going to be young men at the front of the march with their parents, just as last year unilaterally they'd put American war veterans at the front of the march. I had perceived what I thought was a coherent strategy by Stonewall. I suggested it was about time we counteract some of their insidious propaganda. [There] were a series of petty little squabbles over weeks, with letters back and forth in the press. We had said things that allowed people to come out and say what for a long time they had thought. Angela was reported to be in tears and couldn't understand how the community had turned against her. They had no organic links to the community but couldn't stand up to a fight with the likes of us.

STEVE COOK

A new strategy also developed within OutRage! The public dispute between OutRage! and Stonewall, expressed in letters to the gay press and in a series of articles, and the failure of the age of consent campaign, provoked a renewed debate about activism. Further, radical strategies were discussed within the group.

The idea was to freeze OutRage! for a year and to spend a year meeting local groups, training them, developing links, to work for some peak on the run-up to Pride when there'd be a mass media blitz. This idea was shelved, but the spirit was still there.

FERNANDO GUASCH

OutRage! felt it had to make some effort to revitalize its connection with direct action, so we really ought to turn away from Westminster and Parliament and instead go out and see people's local experience in activism, do workshops with them, establish an informal network of people who did direct action. We were aiming to put across some sort of ideology that small-scale direct action should not be allowed to just dwindle.

STEVE COOK

OutRage! was doing a round Britain tour and that was more inspiration. They came up with logos, artwork, and they were inspiring more than anything. It was really good to see people going out and about.

STUART COLLIE

It was very, very, very sad, actually. We found very frightened people, very alienated people, very isolated people, but we didn't find anyone with any spirit to get on and do some actions, other than a small handful who'd identified with us anyway. To my mind, it was very distressing.

STEVE MAYES

It turned out that in all those places where they had lesbian and gay centres, and numbers of professional lesbians and gay men, gravy train and nice jobs, inevitably it was in those places that there'd be complete apathy, people were belligerent, saying we were causing trouble. The places we went to where there was nothing, the whole thing took the tone of a Christian revivalist meeting. People were saying 'Maybe we should... let's book this room next week.' We had a slide show, videos, which people just loved. We came back with charged batteries.

FERNANDO GUASCH

The week-long tour had taken OutRage! to places such as Birmingham, Liverpool and Nottingham, in a minibus full of OutRage! mementoes. In some ways, it was a shrewd move to encourage local grassroots support, and to counter much of the negative publicity OutRage! had been receiving in the national gay and mainstream press. Significantly, though, those OutRage! members who had decided to join the tour were to miss out on a major debate within the group itself, as the running sore of outing reared its head once more.

THIRTEEN

A Right Holy Row

OutRage! zapped Westminster Cathedral (again) after the launch of the new Catholic Catechism on 29 May 1994. Thirteen protesters stood up and raised placards as Cardinal Hume attempted to give a sermon giving his blessing to the new catechism, which claimed that homosexual acts were intrinsically disordered. Riot police were called and escorted the protesters from the Cathedral, although no arrests were made. By the end of the year, attention would shift away from the Catholic Church, and shift squarely to the Church of England in an uncompromisingly confrontational manner.

OutRage!'s traditional 'Queer Heritage' link with Hampstead Heath provided ongoing information as to how the Heath wardens there responded to gay issues as they arose. In July, OutRage! chose to protest at the introduction of a 'trunks on' policy after a ban on nudity at the men's bathing pond on Hampstead. The OutRage! 'strip-off' took place on 10 July after the Corporation of London erected a six-foot high steel wall restricting nude sunbathing to a small enclosure, and imposing a ban on nude sunbathing elsewhere. This was despite a 433 to 247 vote in favour of nude sunbathing taken by pond users the previous year. Although OutRage!'s nude protest raised a few eyebrows, their aim to reverse the ban failed.

Hampstead came under scrutiny again after reports that the Heath wardens were deliberately harassing gay men, and using dogs on site to intimidate cruisers. The persistent reports of intimidation led to a demonstration against the man responsible at the Corporation, Superintendent Paul Canneaux, on 19 August. The specific anti-gay harassment was not the only thing which bothered users of the Heath. A plan to chop down 3000 trees on the West Heath, where much of the gay cruising activity takes place, led to a joint campaign between OutRage! and environmentalist groups, resulting in a climbdown by the Corporation of London.

Queers against fundamentalism

Christian fundamentalism had frequently been a target of OutRage! actions, but reticence had been shown towards actions against other forms of fundamentalism and religious intolerance, particularly against Muslim fundamentalism. Although extremist groups had been targeting student unions and university gay groups for some time threatening violence against lesbian or gay students, the problem had been dealt with largely as one of damage limitation rather than confrontation. However, by 1994, there was increasing publicity of fundamentalist groups such as Hizb-ut-Tahrir, which OutRage! claimed advocated the murder of lesbians and gay men.

In August, Hizb-ut-Tahrir organized a fundamentalist rally at Wembley Arena and, after discussions within OutRage!, a motion to demonstrate at the rally failed to be resolved. Instead, six activists attended a peaceful demonstration under the guise of a group called 'Queers Against Fundamentalism' on 7 August.

The sting in the tail was that we challenged Hizb-ut-Tahrir by identifying them as Nazis, or identifying them with Nazi ideology, the whole thing about genocide, and that went down extremely badly. They argued very powerfully, very coldly, face to face, yes, they wanted to kill me, and it's right that I should be killed. Why could I not accept that? There was no voice of opposition whatsoever.

STEVE MAYES

There was a scam going on in the media about Hizb-ut-Tahrir because they were thought to be associated with terrorism. Hizb-ut-Tahrir were being vilified in the press. I thought it was a bit dodgy to say 'Yeah, yeah, we hate them too, because we're gay.'

SIMON EDGE

Peter and Glenn were arrested and found guilty on the bizarre circumstance that although they were standing in the right place, they caused a group of press photographers to stand in the road. The press caused the obstruction, but Peter and Glen were responsible.

STEVE MAYES

The arrests prompted OutRage! to retrospectively adopt the action and start a campaign fund. Although ordered to pay a £75 fine in January 1995, Tatchell, on a point of principle, refused and was nearly jailed. His appeal was successful and on 9 October 1996 Tatchell won costs. OutRage! claimed that it was a major victory for the right to protest, citing that Peter should not be responsible for the actions of the photographers who had gathered round him and caused an alleged obstruction.

A similar victory was claimed at the 1994 demonstration against the State Opening of Parliament on 16 November. Securing the support of the civil rights group Liberty, OutRage! organized a peaceful demonstration with placards reading 'Equalise Gay Age of Consent Now' and 'Queers demand Equality' as ministers and members of the Royal Family passed by. Given the history of previous actions at State Openings and the fact that this was the first time the police had let a protest take place while the Opening was underway, it was a significant moment and set a precedent not only for gay protests, but civil rights protests generally.

Destabilizing suburbia

Following OutRage!'s interest in and infiltration of the ex-gay movement, information continued to come into the group about the activities of various anti-gay groups. When The Courage Trust planned a meeting for parents of lesbians and gay men at St Andrew's in Chorleywood on 24 September, four activists managed to infiltrate the £7-a-ticket meeting as parents, while others gathered outside.

There was no place to hide in Chorleywood. It is wide boulevards, very quiet. When you get ten queers landing up in that place, what do you do? There was Fernando and Peggy having a huge stand-up row because Peggy was directing us to do one thing and Fernando was saying it was stupid, at which Peter walked off. I thought 'What's going on here? It's supposed to be comrades in arms!'

PHIL JONES

With four people already inside, it was not difficult for the remaining six protesters to barge into the meeting and hand out leaflets containing Lesbian and Gay Switchboard numbers. Eventually, the police were called but made no arrests.

They did a very wonderful thing, which was to take the audience out of the room rather than take us out. When you attack, they always grab the nearest musical instrument and start singing hymns. When they were trying to change pianists, Glenn jumped on the piano stool and started playing Debussy. So the zap finished with all these Christians in tears, all the OutRage! people shouting out loud things like 'Church of hatred, Church of fear, Stop crucifying queers' to this soundtrack of beautiful Debussy, because he's one hell of a pianist. It was surreal.

PHIL JONES

At around the same time, it was revealed that the newly appointed Archbishop of Durham, Michael Turnbull, had been arrested and charged with gross indecency for cottaging in a public toilet in Hull in 1968. Having said that homosexuality was incompatible with a minister's lifestyle earlier in his career, and after finding out that the Church of England hierarchy knew about the conviction, OutRage! began to call for Turnbull's resignation on the grounds that he was a hypocrite.

When Turnbull's enthronement as Archbishop was arranged for 22 October, OutRage! arranged to zap the Bishop. His enthronement and the allegations concerning his cottaging arrest halted a previous plan to 'out' MPs and public figures which had been gathering some steam within OutRage! Instead, a tactical outing was arranged for the night before the Bishop's enthronement.

The night before, at a debate in the Durham Students' Union, I'd been invited to speak in a debate about homosexuality. At my request, Sebastian Sandys, a former Franciscan monk, was invited to speak. At my suggestion, he agreed to out three Anglican bishops who he personally knew to be gay. I primed a selection of journalists to attend the debate with the promise that something sensational would be said about certain bishops. Unfortunately, the debate was late in getting started and by the time Sebastian named names it was already quite late to get his comments into the next day's papers.

PETER TATCHELL

We arrived [in Durham] at exactly the right time. We had to meet Steve Cook at the car park at the station. We were meant to look like we were asking directions or something like that. He said 'Don't look at the car immediately behind, but in it is Joan Bakewell with a camera crew filming!' Somebody was supposed to organize tickets and we'd go in, but they hadn't and we didn't. We changed the plan about four times. Steve was the only one who got arrested beforehand, because he was wearing Doc Martens.

PHIL JONES

We went up to the Cathedral half an hour or so before the new bishop was due to turn up. We weren't sure exactly what we were going to do. There were a lot of police around, more than we expected, and we began to feel they were expecting something. It turns out they were. There was a policeman beside me. When I moved he followed me, so I realized he thought I was suspicious in some way.

DICE

The time came – no Bishop. They changed his procession. There was no way to get at him. Suddenly we heard this eruption and it was Fernando. It was perfect, because by the doorway, there was a whole load of press. All the press started running over. Then we thought we'd got to do something, so we got our placards out and later got into a formation and looked really, really strong. Two seconds later, there was another shout. There was Peter Tatchell running towards the Bishop like some sort of frightened rat, with a placard, and behind him were two coppers.

PHIL JONES

My cue was when Fernando made his dash. That drew all the police attention onto him. At the same time, I darted out of the kitchen door and was able to hurdle the barriers and get onto the green. In the end I got about three-quarters of the way across the green before I was rugby tackled onto the ground by two police officers. I still managed to shout 'The bishop is a hypocrite. He condemns gay people but has had gay sex.' With that the police put their hand across my mouth and stopped me screaming, twisted my arms up my back and started to cart me off.

PETER TATCHELL

It was another nail in the coffin, really. Fucking good action, there were great visuals of a large group of people doing things. Great placard, very simple slogans, but the whole thing focuses on Peter Tatchell. That was the start of the link with Peter Tatchell, that OutRage! are Peter Tatchell's secretariat, his storm-troopers.

PHIL JONES

Although Peter and Fernando were both arrested, neither was charged and there was much publicity around Turnbull's cottaging arrest. However, the action itself did cover up the larger and more radical move made the evening before by Sebastian Sandys – the outing of bishops.

Tell the truth

Although OutRage! had had a non-policy on outing for many years, FROCS had involved OutRage! members and shown a very real belief in the tactics of outing. By the end of 1994, outing had been well and truly established in America and more forceful arguments for its use were being put forward within OutRage!

After Parliament voted against an equal age of consent of 16 for gay men in February, there was a huge groundswell of anger in the gay community. At least 12 of the MPs who voted against 16 were known to be homosexual themselves. This was in our view a clear act of betrayal. That's what put outing back on the agenda in OutRage! There was a long protracted debate over several months. It wasn't until the autumn that we agreed on a new policy, that we would support the outing of people in positions of power and influence who were gay in private but anti-gay in public. In other words, we were targeting their hypocrisy and homophobia – not their homosexuality. Initially in view of the age of consent vote, the people in our sight for outing were the dirty dozen closeted gay MPs who voted against an equal age of consent. We began the process of gathering information. We also decided to compile a list of other public figures for possible targeting including bishops, senior judges, chief constables and military commanders. We would only be satisfied with information that could be corroborated from at least two and preferably four reliable, credible sources.

PETER TATCHELL

What we argued was that outing somebody against their will is a pretty horrible thing to do, and had any one of us been outed, we would have been devastated. But we rationalized it around the concept of self-defence, neutralizing their evil influence on us. So, while we admit it might be morally bad, it's also morally justified because we had to neutralize that person's influence.

FERNANDO GUASCH

I remember planning the tour, and explicitly saying we should not be away for a Thursday meeting, because Peter Tatchell is going to be back, he'll have on the agenda stuff he wants to do. Sure enough, that's what he did. We were late back from Bristol, and he'd got through the meeting an endorsement for the outing campaign.

STEVE COOK

Although we had considerable difficulty in getting cast-iron corroborated evidence about MPs, the information about the closeted gay bishops came to us in torrents. It was eezy peezy. Very quickly, we had the names of ten bishops and the information about them came from reliable, credible sources, mostly from within the Church. It was then just a matter of thinking of an appropriate moment. The opening of the General Synod in November seemed the obvious choice. On the first day we stood there outside as delegates arrived with names of ten bishops on placards with a caption under each one reading 'Tell the truth'. There were also other placards condemning in general terms Anglican homophobia, in particular the support of some Anglican parishes for some anti-gay cults which attempt to cure homosexuals. The response of delegates was a mixture of shock, amusement, incredulity and, from a small minority in the know, surprise that we hadn't named others.

PETER TATCHELL

[It was] probably the least exciting action in terms of what people do that OutRage! has ever done. We had ten people standing there with placards that just said 'Bishop such and such, tell the truth.' It put the cat amongst the pigeons.

PHIL JONES

Within a week, senior church officials were on the phone to the Lesbian and Gay Christian Movement and to OutRage! suggesting a dialogue. The doors that had previously been slammed shut in our faces were suddenly flung wide open. The Lesbian and Gay Christian Movement was asked to submit a discussion document for consideration by the House of Bishops for its next meeting in early January. OutRage! was invited to submit a dossier on homosexual human rights issues, together with our proposals for changes in the law which was also to be presented to the same bishops' meeting. It would never have happened if we had not provoked a crisis in the Church by naming the bishops. Outing really was a catalyst for change. On the evening of the bishops' meeting, at the bishops' request, a delegation of three bishops met with OutRage! for nearly three hours. The bishops' discussion resulted in a public statement deploring anti-gay discrimination and calling on the Church to have a debate about this issue. That was a very important milestone.

PETER TATCHELL

The results have been absolutely dynamic. If ever you need encouragement for outing, this was it. The Church has embraced the issue, has begun the argument in a meaningful way for the first time ever, has appointed a self-confessed 'grey' [see below, pp. 194–5] bishop to the second highest office in the land. If you're afraid of people knowing in the outside world that you're gay, you may not rest safely.

STEVE MAYES

The Lesbian and Gay Christian Movement said we'd achieved in the space of a few weeks what they couldn't achieve in years, which was to get themselves taken seriously.

JOHN JACKSON

Whether the Church of England would have moved on the issues of homosexuality in the Church anyway is debatable – but that it moved quickly afterwards is a matter of fact. Given its suppression of reports recommending a more liberal attitude towards homosexuality, such as the 1988 Osborne Report, it is reasonable to assume that the outing of the bishops, and the press attention on sexuality within the Church, gave a momentum to those advocating change within the Church.

Towards the end of the month, with World AIDS Day looming on 1 December, OutRage! turned its attention once more towards the Roman Catholic Church. On 29 November, they made their way towards Westminster Cathedral, armed with helium-filled condoms and an enormous banner.

We had a military-style operation to invade Westminster Cathedral one morning, release 55 helium-filled condoms and a huge balloon, which flew right up to the ceiling, saying 'Condoms save lives'. That was amazing, it really got them on the defensive. We got them to admit they were killing people by their insistence that people shouldn't use condoms.

JOHN JACKSON

We entered the church, went to the very front, proclaimed who we were, proclaimed our message. We opened the bin bags, let the condoms go up, let the banner go up, it was very successful, you could see it very clearly in the church. One thing happened which we didn't expect, which was that some of the condoms started to burst, and fall on people's faces – an old lady sitting there, and suddenly a condom fell on her. I went back a little later, and the banner was still there. The Church authorities were in the position of having to say why there's a banner saying 'Condoms save lives'! They tried to get a gun from the local police station [to shoot the condoms down], but the police refused to do it.

DICE

OutRage! London was not the only activist group organizing a World AIDS Day demonstration. In Liverpool, OutRage! Merseyside carried out two spectacular zaps.

The first one was outside the Catholic cathedral with a big banner. Two of the group got beaten up by a security guard and chased into the Students' Union building opposite, stuck posters on the glass doors, tied inflated condoms to the railing. We decided to go down to the Albert Dock. I'd learned to fire breathe about six to eight months before, partly out of inspiration from the Lesbian Avengers. We got this impromptu torch and some paraffin, plastered OutRage! banners against the window of 'Richard & Judy' while it was going out. Security come rushing around and I'm fire-breathing this eight-foot flame across the back of the window. Part of it went out [on air].

STUART COLLIE

In late 1994, the Church of England became embroiled in yet another row on gay issues when it became apparent that their charity the Children's Society was the only one of five top children's charities which banned lesbians and gay men from fostering children in their care. The Children's Society ban put it into conflict with government guidelines on good practice, and ignored the recommendations of its own staff working party.

OutRage! wrote to prominent members of the Church of England asking them to comment publicly on issues such as the Children's Society ban on lesbian/gay fostering the bishops' vote against an equal age of consent in the House of Lords, and Church support for anti-gay cults such as the Courage Trust. One of those asked to state their position was John Gladwin, Bishop of Guildford, who declined to comment. He was due to be enthroned as Bishop on 18 December, and the ceremony became a focus for OutRage!'s public attack on the Church of England.

We had to sit with the congregation for a long time in the side aisles. The service was attended by the Chief Constable of Guildford, a lot of dignitaries, very dressed up. I can remember a kid, a little boy, coming up just in front of us and I was talking to him, and my stomach was turning round. At the start of the service, we got up and marched to the front, unfurled our banners and started to shout some slogans. There was a gay priest who was kind of cruising me while we were sitting, and I was cruising him, thinking 'Yeah, he's in for a shock.' In the end, the Chief Constable of Guildford told me he was going to arrest me.

DICE

I knew it was going to be my last zap, so I went totally mad. I'd walked past the musicians, and onto the altar itself, blew fog-horns in his face, threw stinkbombs. We shouted our tits off, fog-horns everywhere. By then, we knew how to swagger and look angry and powerful. I had a workshop on how to look butch. We had the second rule of zapping – you never leave a building vertically, you always leave it horizontally.

FERNANDO GUASCH

We got to a position where we'd got lots more media coverage than ever before. In internal queer politics, OutRage! was perceived to be the main group. Stonewall was nowhere. Anything we did was news. We had endless requests from mainstream TV, mainstream press, wanting to do stuff on OutRage! My view was to get things in the media, get queer stuff in the media, make us visible. It was about fighting back. We're not nice, quiet dinner party homosexuals. We're fuck off queens.

PHIL JONES

At the end of 1994, Peter Tatchell had also gone further with the issues surrounding the outing debate. When the Bishop of London's name, David Hope, had been left off the list of bishops being urged to 'tell the truth', the media expressed surprise. OutRage! argued that for such a prominent Church member, it would be better for him to make up his own mind and talk about his sexuality. As Bishop of London, David Hope was third in the Church of England hierarchy, and in a strong position to influence debates. As the momentum and pressure on the Church of England mounted, Peter decided to take the matter further.

At the end of December I wrote a private letter to David Hope urging him to come out and setting out the reasons why in ethical and practical terms that was the right thing to do. There were no threats or ultimatums in that letter. I made it very clear that this had to be his choice, stressing the tremendous impact that his coming out could have. Precisely so he wouldn't be inadvertently outed if a secretary or assistant read the letter I went to great effort to personally deliver the letter and hand it to him at his residence in Westminster. Although it wasn't my intention, he invited me to come into his study and meet with him. We had a very amicable and friendly 40-minute meeting. At no point did David Hope demur from the suggestion that he was gay. Not once did he intimate that he had been put under pressure. We left on a very warm-hearted note. He saw me to the door and said that he would very carefully consider all the points that I had made and get in touch with me in due course.

PETER TATCHELL

Nothing was heard from the Bishop of London for two months. Wondering if he had come to any decision concerning the issues he had previously discussed over tea, Tatchell contacted David Hope again and asked him if he would communicate his decisions to the group. At the same time, Hope was approached by a journalist who intimated that he was about to be outed by OutRage! The *Independent on Sunday* ran a story about gay clergy in the Church of England, mentioning the Bishop of London in the next sentence. The following day, Hope called a press conference in which he claimed that he'd been put under pressure by OutRage! to come out as gay and felt intimidated into making a public statement. Claiming to be celibate and single all his life, Hope went on to deny being gay but described his own sexuality as a 'slightly grey area'. It was an extraordinary personal statement, but full of criticism of OutRage! and without a positive statement concerning the bishop's own sexuality.

This was not the courageous, confident coming out that OutRage! had wanted. It was half-hearted, messy, ambiguous and filled with bitter recriminations. Nevertheless, it was a tacit admission that the third most senior bishop in the Church of England had a homosexual component, was at least in part homosexual. We'd succeeded in getting him to come out, albeit half-heartedly. Even better, we'd done it in a way that forced the Church to rally round him in support. The last thing we'd have wanted was for him to be isolated, condemned, forced out the Church. The world conference of Anglican primates which coincidentally happened to be meeting in Britain at the time issued a statement of solidarity and called on the Church to rethink their attitude on homosexuality. This was a fantastic achievement. It was all we had hoped for come true.

PETER TATCHELL

Peter wrote to the Bishop on an OutRage! letterhead saying we think it would be good for you to come out and this struck me as just blackmail. You have just outed ten bishops, how can you pretend you're just giving this person moral advice? When the Bishop called our bluff by making his letter public, I think the honourable thing would have been to perhaps say 'Well, this bugger deserves to be outed.' But instead, Peter fucked it up totally and made a fool of himself by going to the press and saying we didn't threaten him at all. We had a very easy to understand moral line and we should have stuck to it.

FERNANDO GUASCH

Subsequently, the Archbishop of Canterbury instigated the establishment of a bishop's sexuality group which has begun a wide-ranging review of Church policy on lesbian and gay issues including dialogue with lesbian and gay community organizations. The witch-hunting of parish priests seems more or less to have ended. It opened up greater acceptance of gay priests, resulting in a number of individuals feeling able to come out for the first time. All in all, the naming of the bishops and the attempt to persuade David Hope have been tremendously positive. Outing has been a catalyst for reform within the Church of England.

PETER TATCHELL

FOURTEEN

Homosexual Terrorists Kill MP

Having gathered information on homosexual Members of Parliament, OutRage! set about drawing up a plan of action for using it. OutRage! were not the only group who picked up information on closeted gay people in public life – both Stonewall and the Lesbian and Gay Christian Movement had formal and informal sources of information on who might be gay. That OutRage! was the first gay group to publicly make use of this information set it apart as a group of 'homosexual terrorists' in the eyes of the media.

The move towards outing MPs gathered force in January 1995, as OutRage! drew up a list of MPs they would write a letter to, inviting them to 'come out'. Twenty MPs from a cross-section of four political parties were sent letters, posted first class on 28 January and sent by recorded delivery. The names of the MPs were not issued by OutRage!, although a press release containing a copy of the letter sent (with identifying features blanked out) was issued. The letter, marked 'STRICTLY PRIVATE & CONFIDENTIAL. Sensitive Personal Information. For the Eyes of the MP Only [sic]', did not threaten to out the MPs, but urged them to come out voluntarily.

OutRage! has received information which suggests that you may be gay or bisexual. This information comes from sources which we believe to be reliable and credible...we urge you...to make the morally responsible choice to come out voluntarily.[1]

After outlining many of the reasons why positive role models can be important for young lesbians and gay men, and giving reassurance that coming out might be more daunting in theory than in practice, the letter cited the example of Chris Smith as an out gay MP, and made reference to Prime Minister John Major's statement that being gay was no bar to holding a ministerial position in his government. It continued:

The dishonesty of closeted gay MPs corrodes the integrity of public life and diminishes public respect for Parliament. Many people will rightly ask: if an MP is not being truthful about their sexuality, what else are they not being truthful about? The vast majority of voters respect honesty and the potential loss of votes from a declining number of bigots is likely to be outweighed by the support of broad minded electors.

Coming out removes the stress of leading a double life and removes the fear of exposure by political opponents and the press. Secrecy and sexual dishonesty offer great opportunities for the media to sensationalise an MP's private life. Being open allows gay MPs to lead honest and dignified lives and denies the press the scope for scandal-mongering.

As Michael Brown MP has recently stated, 'coming out' has lifted a great psychological burden. The adverse consequences he feared have not materialised. He now wishes he had come out a long time ago. MPs contemplating coming out may wish to consider doing so with several of their colleagues, thus removing the possibility of an individual being a target of the tabloids. Once there are several openly gay MPs in Parliament, voters will judge them on their policies, not on their sexual orientation. Coming out is empowering and fulfilling. *It is the ethically right thing to do.*

[Name of MP] you have a duty to yourself for your peace of mind, as well as a moral obligation to other lesbians and gay men, to be open about your sexuality . We wish you the personal strength and courage to live your life with openness, honesty and integrity.

Yours sincerely
OutRage![2]

Every time we start off, we start off with a good idea and it gets watered down and watered down and watered down. We just asked them to be honest, and because it comes from OutRage!, it's got a certain risk to it. We said anybody who voted for 16, who didn't vote for section 28, your private life is your private life, unless you do something to harm the gay community, in which case you're a vicious bastard who needs to be neutralized. There were two Ulster Unionists, and it included two Cabinet Ministers. We did all sorts of stupid things like making sure they were inside an envelope inside an envelope inside another, so the secretaries didn't open it. We were adamant that we wouldn't under any circumstances say who was on the list, publicly.

PHIL JONES

Apparently, he [Peter Tatchell] could not see that it could be perceived as a threat by the recipients. I was given a list – not by OutRage! – which I think was accurate, in the sense that it was the one OutRage! had sent. I don't think it was accurate in terms of sexuality.

SIMON EDGE

The letter was sent out ... And it was ignored, totally. Until the bishop's thing, when outing was in the news – Peter somehow had the idea of re-press releasing the letter, which he did, and by lunchtime of that day, we had a bit of a snowball on our hands. There was a motion in the House of Commons condemning it, people being very indignant.

JOHN JACKSON

No politician came out, or contacted OutRage!, and the original letter didn't become a news story. However, following publicity over the Bishops' meeting to discuss homosexuality in early 1995, a new momentum around sexuality took over. In an interview for BBC TV's *Westminster On Line* in March, Peter Tatchell drew attention to the letter sent two months earlier. Suddenly, there was considerable interest in the 'outing letter', but from an unexpected source. The *Belfast Telegraph* somehow got hold of information that James Kilfedder, a Unionist MP, was one of those people on the list. Talking to Peter in the OutRage! office, without naming the MP involved, a journalist asked a series of cryptic questions to attempt to determine the identity of a recipient of the letter.

I think possibly the one mistake that was made was that Peter gave hints. When the Press rang up and said 'What parties have you sent them out to?' he mentioned one of the Ulster parties. They said which one, and there's only two or three, and he said it was the small one, which you can count the number of MPs on one hand. And that's how a lot of the press cottoned on to James Kilfedder.

JOHN JACKSON

The *Belfast Telegraph* rang James Kilfedder to say 'we believe you've received a letter from OutRage! alleging you're gay'. The first editions come out, by which time James Kilfedder is on a plane to Gatwick, so he hasn't seen the paper then. Lands at Gatwick, gets on the Gatwick Express and between Gatwick and Victoria he has a heart attack and dies. Then there was the Siege of Bermondsey.

PHIL JONES

The *Belfast Telegraph* had published a headline 'Hardline Gay Group Targets Ulster MP' on Monday 20 March, just before Ulster Popular Unionist Party

MP Sir James Kilfedder, a hardline anti-gay MP, died from a heart attack. The following morning, the *Daily Mirror*'s front-page article carried the headline 'Gay Slur Riddle of Sudden Death MP'. Other papers also began to speculate that OutRage!'s alleged threat to out an Ulster MP may have caused Kilfedder's death.

I remember I got back from work and there was this very, very scared phone call from Peter Tatchell saying 'What shall I do? I'm sitting in the dark. I've got the press at my front door. I've got my phone ringing all the time.' When the news got out about the *Belfast Telegraph*, everyone was just really, really fucked off. Up until then, we'd been in control of what was happening. We'd been pushing the press and suddenly they turned on us. It was massive. If they wanted to, they could get into every single person's private life. The *Daily Telegraph* had someone in Melbourne going through Peter Tatchell's mother's bin!

PHIL JONES

They seized upon us as terrorists, sexual terrorists, blackmailers, fascists, sexual storm-troopers, Peter as the devil himself. That was extremely upsetting for us all. The letter he'd written was shown up on the news and the address was visible. Of course, he had Combat 18[3] and others visiting him. As a result of this, they also said that we were blackmailing these 20 MPs. That caused a lot of trouble within the group – we were exhausted emotionally and things got confused.

MARINA CRONIN

Peter was the most hated man in Britain. The effect on the group was awful, because a small number of people were involved in OutRage!, punch drunk after the success of the bishops' action, suddenly find themselves under sustained and fierce attack from the press and they didn't know how to handle it. The group cracked. Suddenly everyone was running for cover saying 'This isn't what we meant to do', going into this denial tactic as a means of defence. There were about three or four people who were staffing the phones and answering enquiries and increasingly because a lot of those people had very little experience, a number of gaffs were made. A number of statements were made which were damaging, stupid, dangerous, but absolutely understandable. People started looking around internally for a scapegoat, and of course the scapegoat more than ever was Peter.

STEVE MAYES

Someone who's not a member of OutRage! decided they were going to out [two cabinet ministers] at the same time. We got him onto

Newsnight, where he was going to do it. Peter phoned up *Newsnight* and said 'No, I'll come on instead.' At that point, we could have gone ballistic, in terms of queer politics, because it was all about Cabinet Ministers. We know they've got pictures, but they won't run them, for reasons of their own. With one more push, we could have blown the whole thing open. We were all very stressed. It ended in a huge, huge row in the office. Fernando was [brought] in. That was the most horrendous thing I've ever seen in terms of personal demolitions. I think a lot of stuff that Fernando had wanted to say to Peter for a long time just came out.

PHIL JONES

Here was somebody trading on the name of an organization that had been going a long time, which had a good reputation, who was absolutely unaccountable. So I did a telephone survey in *Capital Gay*, 'Peter – Prince or Prat', and it came out about 50:50. I didn't think it was innately conservative to say, 'Hang on, you're a loose cannon.' There are twin assumptions. In the outside world, there's an assumption that OutRage! is Peter. As a consequence, in the gay community, people thought OutRage! was lots of people, it wasn't Peter, and they held to that even when it wasn't true. Even if other people come to the meeting, he's one of the oldest and the most eloquent, puts in all the work, so you can have the bullshit about not having an El Presidente, but it is a one-man band.

SIMON EDGE

The Kilfedder death brought to the fore many of the debates about who ran OutRage! and who was making decisions. Ever since the outing of the bishops, OutRage! had dominated headlines on gay issues and led the debate. Outing was a tough issue, and the publicity around a death associated with OutRage! was enough to pressurize a small, hard-worked group of volunteers. But on the death of James Kilfedder MP, OutRage! were unrepentant:

Why should we feel sorry about the death of a bigoted MP? Anyone like Kilfedder who victimises the lesbian and gay community will get no sympathy from us.[4]

February saw the anniversary of the 1994 age of consent vote, where so much hope, energy and reason had been lost. The outing issue had become significant because of the information OutRage! received on those 'dirty dozen' gay MPs who had voted against an equal age of consent, and even before the death of Kilfedder, the outing of MPs, and the names of those gay MPs, were common knowledge within and outside OutRage!

We were talking about what to do for the 21st February anniversary and there was talk of the dirty dozen MPs, outing them, and that was quite controversial, people weren't sure. Although we had reliable proof, the witnesses weren't prepared to stand up in court 'cause they'd lose their jobs. Everybody knew – within the meeting it was quite clear who the twelve were. It wasn't as much kept a secret as not talked about. It was talked about openly at the Tuesday meeting.

MARINA CRONIN

For the anniversary of the vote on the age of consent, OutRage! opted for a less radical event than a high-profile outing campaign, and called a rally and vigil for 21 February.

As it happened, it was a bitterly cold night. There were something like 700–800 of us, we had candles, fog-horns, whistles. The Sisters of Perpetual Indulgence were there. Some people were queuing to lobby MPs, that was our excuse for being there. There was meant to be one or two minutes of silence to remember the victims of the age of consent laws and queerbashing.

MARINA CRONIN

It was the first time I'd seen the Sisters manifested anywhere, with Mother Molesta walking up and down with the holy water. Quite a few people got in to lobby MPs, but there wasn't the sense of occasion of the first year. It was good to mark the occasion, but it was a non-event.

STUART COLLEY

Bashing the bishops (again)

After OutRage! Merseyside had 'conferred' with a delegation of bishops in early 1995, one member managed to infiltrate the offices of the ex-gay cult the True Freedom Trust at one of their bases in Liverpool.

I found out there was an HIV charity, a service provider in Liverpool called CASIA – stands for Care Against Sufferers from AIDS or something like that, something that sounded sensible. On their Board of Trustees was someone from the True Freedom Trust, a bloke called Martin Allet. I did a bit of work, writing to the main funders of the True Freedom Trust, and people would come along to the OutRage! meeting with information about it. CASIA got closed down which I'm really pleased about because they were referring people to the True Freedom

Trust. I started going to CASIA, had an interview with the director to discuss my concerns. I met this bloke and talked to him about the True Freedom Trust and he said that the True Freedom Trust were OK even though they're linked in with Exodus and loads of other international ex-gay movements.

The day I went for the meeting I went over and I came up with this fake name, Mark Collins. Half-way through this interview, which was going quite well, this bloke from CASIA walks in that I'd been going to see two or three weeks before and looked at me and went 'Oh, hello, what are you doing here?' At which point Martin Allett looked at the bloke and said 'Do you know each other? You're from OutRage! aren't you?' At which point I picked up my coat and ran out the door, rumbled and freaked.

STUART COLLIE

OutRage! London managed to infiltrate the True Freedom Trust much more successfully, with one member regularly attending meetings. When the TFT planned to hold a large recruitment meeting in July, OutRage!'s mole quickly fed back the information and a zap was set up for the small Baptist Church in Westbourne Park where the meeting was scheduled for 21 July.

There was a guy from the organization who was sitting in a chair between the two rooms. When he saw us all, he tried to block our way. We managed to get into one of the rooms. They were sitting in there talking about God. We engaged in conversation with a lot of these people. I remember one guy was very angry, he kept tearing at everything we had. I was talking to someone for ages, about my religious background, trying to convince him of the naturalness of homosexuality, and I felt I was getting somewhere.

DICE

One guy was about 70, others in their twenties... Some of the people were shouting at us to get out, devils, obviously terrified of us because we were what they were trying to get rid of in themselves. I remember Martin Corbett was talking to somebody who was looking out the window the whole time, who started crying. I had to zap Josh, who was our mole, which was quite difficult. We found out a couple of people had walked out. The True Freedom Trust had lost three or four people, we'd saved them from that.

MARINA CRONIN

The next day, OutRage! had planned yet another zap against the Church of England. The Bishop of St Albans, the Rt Rev John Taylor, had been a supporter of ex-gay group the Courage Trust, who had operated from out of his diocese for a number of years. John Taylor had refused to comment publicly on the matter on a number of occasions. On 22 July, he was due to give a sermon at his farewell service in St Albans Cathedral.

There had been numerous attempts – letter-writing, phone calls – to talk to the Bishop and explain the situation. He refused to listen, once he actually slammed the phone down on us. We thought, enough is enough, we're going to say goodbye to him in a way which we feel is appropriate. We turned up at his Cathedral and it was full of people. We had to sit through these diabolical hymns and prayers, all of us in straight drag, with newspapers under our arms. He got up to speak. Glenn popped up and immediately started saying 'This is a peaceful OutRage! protest', exposing the Courage Trust and how the Bishop refused to do anything. All the rest of us went to the front and stood with our placards. Dice managed to get up on the pulpit and was wheeled off screaming and shouting. At one point the microphone was left on and he was chanting 'Church of hatred, Church of fear, Stop crucifying queers!' through the microphone. The Church people, stewards, were quite violent towards us, they were really pushing us. I had a whistle round my throat which was yanked backwards.

MARINA CRONIN

Dice was behind him with a placard, and he said to Dice, 'Can I leave please?' and Dice said 'Yes, of course' and so he did. They then proceeded to move the pulpit, which was on wheels with Dice still inside it holding this placard. It was a really Monty Python moment, it was so funny. I think it was on that occasion Martin Corbett – when somebody came up to him and was being very aggressive – turned to them and said 'Oh, get away, you've got bad breath!'

JOHN JACKSON

Since then, the new Bishop of St Albans, we contacted him and he made it a top priority to have a meeting with us. That was January of [1996]. Stuart, John Jackson and myself met him and talked for about an hour and a half. He was quite supportive, sympathetic. We got on quite well with him. [The Courage Trust] have stopped their residential courses, where people have to pay.

MARINA CRONIN

The Courage Trust were only part of a much wider picture within the ex-gay movement. Having built up a network of sources about the groups, OutRage! continued to feed information to the gay and mainstream press, generating a public debate about the ex-gay movement. In August, the target of OutRage!'s first action against the ex-gay movement, St Michael's Church in Belgravia, played host to an international conference being held by the Living Waters group. The conference, on 23 August 1995, was visited by OutRage! four years after their first protests at the Church.

We had our mole from the True Freedom Trust zap, one of the stewards. He had tickets with false names, badges for people. A number of people managed to get into the church, all armed with placards and stink bombs, but not enough stink bombs as it turned out. Then a whole lot of other people burst in with fog-horns, made a complete racket, and there were more people outside. We crucified Sarah, wearing an OutRage! T-shirt, on a wonderful pink crucifix, with a wreath of daffodils on her head.

MARINA CRONIN

Shortly after the zap, the ITV documentary *The Big Story* exposed the ex-gay movement, and resulted in at least one of its leaders, Chris Metcalf, resigning from the London True Freedom Trust following allegations that he sexually molested young gay men. The documentary featured footage from many of OutRage!'s demonstrations and widened the debate and concern over the operation of ex-gay 'therapy' and counselling within the Church of England, which was forced to distance itself from such groups.

In October of the same year, OutRage! – with the help of *Gay Times* journalist Vicky Powell – researched the background to some of the ex-gay organizations to discover who funded them. The Jerusalem Trust, a substantial shareholder in J. Sainsbury PLC and one of the Sainsbury family trusts, had given over £22,000 to the True Freedom Trust over the previous two years. Trustees included the Conservative MP for Hove, Tim Sainsbury, and the Conservative MP for Finchley, Hartley Booth. With the Lesbian Avengers, OutRage! staged a picket of Sainsbury's in Camden Town, London on 1 October. Later, they also organized an action at the Sainsbury Wing of the National Gallery.

Our original aim was to urge people not to shop at Sainsbury. That was quite a difficult action to do, because everyone shops there! The National Gallery, Sainsbury's Wing. Ten or 12 Lesbian Avengers handcuffed themselves on the main stairs, the ones at each end were handcuffed to the railings. A security guard marched up through the line and knocked over one of the Avengers whose handcuffs broke with the force and she was then taken off to hospital with cuts and bruises.

MARINA CRONIN

On 27 November, Peter Tatchell and other members of OutRage! took their complaints directly to the Church of England on the eve of the opening session of the General Synod. Their protest symbolically echoed Martin Luther's 1517 protest in Wittenberg when he nailed his 'Ninety-Five Theses Against Indulgences' against a church door and started the Reformation.

We rushed the door, they closed the door on us – we kicked the shins of one of the security guards who was closing the door on us. The police took 15 minutes to arrive. Parliament Square, defacing an ancient monument – and the police took 15 minutes to get there. We closed the front doors. Molly was charged with the responsibility of lifting the bolts and as it was my first action in London, I was amazed at the organization that had gone into it. To see all the work put into it beforehand, the organization, the way it was all choreographed, everyone had roles, even down to choosing the shape and the size of the nail, this big antique, handmade, six-inch nail was used... looking at the hole in the door beforehand so we couldn't be done for criminal damage.

STUART COLLEY

We made this beautiful-looking list. We nailed that onto the door. It did fall off at one point, but we managed to get it on. The same day, it was 25 years since the first GLF demo at Highbury Fields. All the activist groups joined together to remember that, with a candle-lit vigil. We all went to the pub which used to be called the Cock Tavern where the GLF used to meet.

MARINA CRONIN

The list of demands was titled 'Four Theses Against Church Homophobia', calling for a 'Queer Reformation':

We the queer victims of Anglican homophobia call on the Church to cease its support for anti-gay discrimination:

† Stop persecuting openly gay clergy in honest and loving relationships

† End the Children's Society ban on lesbian and gay foster parents

† Withdraw support from anti-gay cults which attempt to 'cure' queers of their sexuality

† Sack the Bishops in the House Of Lords who voted against an equal age of consent[5]

The call for a 'Queer Reformation' neatly summed up some of the key demands which OutRage! had been fighting against the Church of England over during the previous six years. Emphasising the Church's moral duty to preserve the rights of lesbians and gay men and end endorsement of anti-gay discrimination focused media attention and public debate on how the Church of England dealt with the issue of sexuality, which is still ongoing.

NOTES

1. Letter to MPs from OutRage!, 27 January 1995.
2. Letter to MPs, January 1995.
3. Combat 18 are a neo-Nazi organization taking their name from the position of Adolf Hitler's initials in the alphabet. As well as the predictable anti-Semite and racist views they express, they have a strong homophobic stand, as graffiti close to me in Coventry testifies.
4. Quote attributed to OutRage!, 'Heart attack MP was sent "outing" letter', the *Pink Paper*, 24 March 1995.
5. OutRage! Press Release – 'GAYS NAIL DEMANDS TO WESTMINSTER ABBEY DOOR', 27 November 1995.

FIFTEEN

The Death of Activism?

By 1995 OutRage! had developed a different focus and different tactics to combat homophobia. Smaller numbers in the group had meant a slicker, more contained group, but one which could not sustain large-scale zaps or large participatory events as in the early 1990s. OutRage! began to concentrate on intervening in debates, national and international, using their reputation as a radical group to deliver controversial arguments as an antidote to the more assimilationist mood of the expanded London gay scene.

More urgently, by 1995 OutRage! was having to make appeals for funds in order to keep its offices at Peter Street. With an annual bill of £2500 for the office rent, OutRage! set about contacting sympathetic groups and individuals to persuade them to donate money and support.

OutRage! is one of the most effective lesbian and gay campaigning groups. This is achieved despite massive under-resourcing. Our total annual budget is a mere £8,000 (compared to £200,000 for Stonewall and £100,000 for Lesbian & Gay Employment Rights). We are not only effective politically, but cost-effective as well.

OutRage! could achieve even more if we had secure and regular campaign funding. We don't have a much-needed photocopier, mobile phone or internet connection, and we lack many basic office facilities, such as a heater for the winter months.

OutRage! receives no funding from benefactors or foundations. Our finances are based on the exhausting and time-consuming shaking of collection tins in pubs and clubs – which constantly diverts our energies from the priority of campaigning...

OutRage! has a positive, proven record of commitment and achievement. We hope that with your generous financial support we will be able to continue and strengthen our financial efforts for lesbian, gay and bisexual emancipation.[1]

The appeal was successful – OutRage! managed to gain enough money to pay its bills and more, so that its financial crisis became a successful show of support for its aims and objectives. Although the biggest donations remained anonymous, at least two major gay stars donated large amounts to keep the group and its ideas alive.

Wreaths and Queen's Balls

The calling of a Rally for Islam by Hizb-ut-Tahrir – the same group which Queers Against Fundamentalism had demonstrated against the previous year – launched OutRage! into another campaign against Muslim fundamentalism. They planned a demonstration for the day of the rally, 13 August.

They'd organized this Rally for Islam in Trafalgar Square, where they were expecting thousands of people to attend. In fact, only about 2000 people attended. We turned up, invited lots of other groups such as Lesbian Avengers, Stonewall, Jewish groups. We wanted to stand outside Canada House, which would have been right near, but were moved on by police. We stood instead on the other side of the road. We had our fog-horns and whistles and banners and placards. It didn't go quite according to plan – we were meant to have a pink tank, like GMFA had at Pride. We had hired that, arranged to pay for it. The day before, they let us down at the last minute.

MARINA CRONIN

OutRage! was also in contact with a TV company which had been following Islamic Fundamentalist leader Omar Bakri Mohammad, and was feeding it information. The Muslim extremist group Al-Muhajiroun had originally planned to hold an enormous rally at Wembley Arena, at which OutRage! would demonstrate.

London Arena were getting concerned it would get a little hairy. We weren't hiding the fact that we were going to do this demonstration. Word obviously gets back to the organizers, and London Arena, fearing a mass protest outside, decide they'd need more security and the security costs went up by 40 per cent which apparently Al-Muhajiroun could not afford. I think they were planning all along to get loads of publicity. What happened was that the rally got cancelled but they decided to have the press conference at Speaker's Corner. So we thought, right, we'll go as well to Speaker's Corner, it's not that much hassle.

STUART COLLEY

On 8 September, OutRage! confronted the Saudi dissident Dr Muhammad Al-Mass'ari and Omar Bakri Mohammad in Hyde Park. Claiming that Al-Muhajiroun incite hatred against Jews, homosexuals and Hindus, OutRage! quoted from an Al-Muhajiroun leaflet titled 'Homosexuality, Bestiality, Lesbianism, Adultery and Fornication' which claimed that homosexual relations were a 'crime against humanity' and boasted that Islam advocates the death penalty for homosexuality. OutRage! declared a 'Queer Jihad' against Islamic fundamentalism, judging Omar Bakri Mohammad guilty of crimes against queer humanity and issuing a 'Queer Fatwa' condemning him to 1000 years of relentless sodomitical torture.

As soon as we swept up with the pink banners and flags the media just turned away from Omar Bakri and the police were trying to divide us. We were on one side of Speaker's Corner, they were on another. Peter managed to have a discussion with Dr Al-Mass'ari, the darling of the liberal community, under threat of deportation from Britain. I got into a debate. I've got my arms draped around my boyfriend and surrounded by groups of Islamic supporters, a circle of photographers and police and I'm stood opposite Omar Bakri arguing the toss about religious theory, his interpretation of God's words, the most bizarre conversation. I'm feeling the top of his shoulders, at the top of his arm, which is giving me the biggest sexual thrill that I've had in years and I'm stood there opposite this homophobic cunt.

STUART COLLEY

Following anti-gay comments by Zimbabwe's President Mugabe in early 1995, OutRage! allied itself with an international campaign against anti-gay sentiment and legislation in Zimbabwe. Ironically this was part of the same campaign as Amnesty International, whom they had zapped only four years previously over their refusal to adopt gay prisoners of conscience. OutRage! then planned a zap outside the Zimbabwe High Commission in London on 18 July.

It was a joint demonstration with GALZ (Gays And Lesbians of Zimbabwe), Stonewall, Lesbian Avengers. That action was simultaneous with an action in Harare. We gathered outside the Zimbabwe High Commission with placards. The news about Zimbabwe in 1996 is that the Zimbabwe HIV/AIDS forum was launched in London and Peter Tatchell and myself went to that and Peter spoke to the High Commissioner in London and asked if a meeting could be arranged with OutRage! and GALZ to talk about how they're going to have this HIV/AIDS forum without gay rights in Zimbabwe and the High Commissioner did agree to a meeting.

MARINA CRONIN

Echoing an early action when the group was in its fledgling days in 1990, on 12 November 1995, Remembrance Day, OutRage! organized the laying of a pink wreath at the Cenotaph to remember lesbian and gay victims of the Holocaust and those lesbian and gay civilians and military personnel who died fighting Nazism. Also sponsored by the Jewish Lesbian and Gay Helpline and the Gay and Lesbian Humanist Association, the event was organized to draw attention to the plight of survivors of the concentration camps. Because they had been branded as 'common criminals' or 'sexual perverts', many gay survivors were denied compensation, while the years spent in the camps were subtracted from their pension entitlements. OutRage! also claimed that no Nazi doctors had been prosecuted for medical experiments conducted on gay inmates, which included castration and hormonal implants. To add poignancy to the event, OutRage! invited 72-year-old Jewish lesbian Sharley McClean to lay the wreath alongside 16-year-old OutRage! member Marina Cronin. McClean's uncle had been arrested following a Gestapo raid on a gay cabaret club in Berlin in 1937, and died in Sachsenhausen concentration camp, where he had been forced to wear the pink triangle badge to denote that he was a homosexual. McClean's socialist father was also arrested and beaten to death, while her mother had also died in a camp. McClean had been rescued and came to Britain as a refugee child in 1939.

We made the wreath ourselves, pink carnations, beautiful. I think we laid our wreath after the Salvation Army and before the National Front. Rather nice timing! The whole idea of that action was to highlight the fact that it's often ignored in history books that a huge amount of gay people, particularly gay men, were killed, just like the Jews were. That was a fact that was hidden or denied by people. We wanted people to hear this fact and to understand that we were honouring these people, trying to remember them. We had originally discussed other ideas for that action. There was talk about interrupting the minute's silence with fog-horns or something. Some people felt we should do it, others felt the minute's silence is a respectful thing, it would hurt people. We decided against that.

MARINA CRONIN

The sombre tone of the Cenotaph wreath was in stark contrast to a later action at the end of the year. Every year, the Queen holds a Royal Ball for her members of staff. Previously, she had reportedly been outraged that same-sex partners had been showing affection to each other at the parties, so in 1995 a circular was issued with the Ball invites disallowing gay male partners. The information had been sent to Peter Tatchell from a contact who was a member of the Royal Staff.

We decided to go along in drag, do a pantomime-type travesty outside. The banners were fantastic, like pennant shaped banners, with the 'Wicked Witch of Windsor' and 'Good Queen Betty Stands Exposed'.

I managed to borrow this fantastic dress, lent to me by Julian Howes. It was the first time I'd done drag in public. The dress was made for the Latin section of 'Come Dancing'. It was bright orange and black, with false skirt and loads and loads of netting underneath it. I remember being so panic-stricken. So there I am valiumed out of my face, dragged up to the nines, walking from the OutRage! office down to Piccadilly tube, arrangements of netting, going down the escalators in Piccadilly Circus with a bank of photographers at the bottom.

STUART COLLEY

Of all the actions that we had done that year, that had to be the least important of all. That got the most coverage. It was absolutely pissing down with rain. We had our pennants with funny slogans on – 'What's a ball without fairies'. It was Martin Corbett's last action. He wasn't very well at the time, he went along in his Saint Wizard outfit.

MARINA CRONIN

Newsnight turned up for it. They were doing this interview with me dragged up, make-up running half way down my face and this drop of water on the end of my nose, and they actually broadcast. There were lots of upset and outraged members of staff and also some quite supportive. I believe nine members of staff stayed away in protest.

STUART COLLEY

Queer Cupid and bloody cute fluffy animals

By the start of 1996, OutRage! had gone cyber and had its own Web page on the Internet which included information, press releases and photographs.

It was also a way to disseminate information about new campaigns to a potential audience of hundreds of thousands of people internationally. When OutRage! launched its first major campaign of 1996, around the age of consent, it already had briefing documents available on the World Wide Web. Shifting the debate away from a simple call for equality at 16, OutRage! demanded that the age of consent itself should be brought down to 14 for both heterosexuals and homosexuals, launching the campaign at the Houses of Parliament on the eve of St Valentine's Day, 13 February. With Queer Cupid and companions bearing huge Valentine's cards, OutRage! claimed that an age of consent at 14 would bring Britain in line with 20 other European countries. OutRage! also demanded that sex involving young people below the age of consent at 14 should not be prosecuted if both partners consent, and there were no more than three years' difference in their ages – similar to German, Swiss and Israeli law. OutRage! also called for better sex education in schools, to reduce the incidence of sexual abuse, pregnancies, abortions and sexually transmitted diseases.

The campaign was really a press campaign, just to get the issue aired. We had decided that the age of consent had to be equal, but there was more mileage in talking about an age of consent of perhaps 14 because two thirds of gay men have sex before the age of 16, one third of lesbians, a lot of straights. We thought 16 wasn't really in touch with what young people are really doing. Rob Collins was dressed up as Cupid and we had our placards in the shape of hearts. It got quite a wide airing. There was never a question that we would get an age of 14, it was more of an idea, to wake people up, not to agree with everyone else. We felt that the age of consent debate had died. We thought the only way people will start talking about it again is to do something radical.

MARINA CRONIN

The group was starting to lose it a bit. We'd lost a lot of members and [we were] basically a skeletal set of people, the most prominent being Peter, with very little opposition. Peter was getting it all his own way and had some strange ideas, stuff that in themselves I tend to agree with, but the timing of it and the politics of it I think are completely inappropriate, and wrong for OutRage! to be taking on board. It wasn't about equality, it was about empowering people to take control of their sex lives and stop criminalizing people under the age of consent. I disagreed with it at the time and to a certain extent I disagree with it now. It caused a lot of furore and upset a lot of people that didn't need upsetting. We need to get an equal age of consent first before we start putting ourselves up as targets for the usual arguments.

STUART COLLEY

OutRage! also used the issue in a debate in the Houses of Parliament organized by the National Union of Students, where panel speakers included Chris Smith, Angela Mason and Edwina Currie. The call for an age of consent at 14 did initiate controversy and debate within the gay community, and reminded the wider world that the law was still discriminating against young gay men.

By March, OutRage! had returned to one of its original campaigning issues: queerbashing and the police. A gay man, Rory Green, had been arrested for defending himself and his HIV-positive partner against a violent queerbashing. In an attempt to defend himself against his assailant Adonis Alan, Green had hit him with a champagne bottle he was carrying. Green was charged with grievous bodily harm, while the assailant had his charges reduced from affray to common assault and criminal damage, with two years' conditional discharge and a £50 fine for compensation. Previously, the local police had refused to act on complaints of serious threats from the same attacker. On 2 March, OutRage! took their protest directly to Fulham Police Station.

We decided that we were going to do a stencil on the ground of a body in spray paint and then… Queers Bash Back… right next to the steps of Fulham Police Station. There was hardly anyone there. Peter absented himself. Phil Jones was very nervous about the whole situation and just before we were about to go up there, Phil got a sort of panic attack and said 'I don't think I can do this, I'm concerned about the way this is going. I'm getting this tunnel vision, I can't see anything.' We went round the corner and we'd got these luminous distress flares that went bright red and gave out loads of smoke. We marched up, David Kitchen's lying on the floor so we spray painted round David Kitchen, as they're letting off these marine distress flares which are giving out loads of bright red light. Just as I'm finishing off the Queers Bash Back stencil, this copper appears and is forced to arrest me. I've got the release form which came a couple of weeks later and a hand-written note on the bottom saying 'NB Hammersmith & Fulham Council will be contacting you regarding the cleaning costs'.

STUART COLLEY

OutRage! caused further controversy when it officially sent a letter to a US march against animal testing, claiming that animals should not be used for tests of experimental drugs or vaccines even where fatal human infections such as HIV were concerned. Orthodox gay politics at the time was claiming that animal experiments were justified in order to end human suffering. OutRage! claimed that no major advance in AIDS treatment had been made through the use of animals in experiments, and that such experiments were a waste of resources. At the US March for the Animals in Washington DC on 23 June, British rock star Chrissie Hynde read out OutRage!'s letter of support:

We do not believe that the oppression of queer people can or should be remedied by the oppression of other peoples or species.

Even when faced with the horror of the AIDS epidemic, there can be no ethical justification for colluding with the victimisation of living, thinking, feeling creatures.

It is a moral outrage that in the name of stopping HIV, some people are prepared to condone the wilful infliction of suffering on sentient beings, such as chimpanzees and monkeys, which clearly experience physical pain and emotional distress as a result of HIV-related experiments conducted upon them.

As queer people who have suffered victimisation, we feel a special responsibility to speak out for all animals, human and non-human, who suffer violations of their dignity and rights.[2]

You can't afford to make a lesbian and gay movement tied to what is in effect a sectarian issue, or a matter of conscience. The claims that animal experimentation is always wrong is one I'd contest. I actually believe there is much evidence of humane experiments which have real benefits, not least of which is to people with HIV or AIDS. You wouldn't have protease inhibitors without animal experimentation. People who deny that are scientifically inaccurate.

SIMON WATNEY

I'm like 'What the fuck had this got to do with queer issues, what has this got to do with fighting homophobia?' Basically, it's one of Peter's little babies that really I don't think is an OutRage! issue. I don't think it falls within the stated aims, I think it's sentimental and ill thought out. I think we've really shot ourselves in the foot on it, yet we received massive world-wide publicity from it which to me is amazing. Queers are being bashed in the streets, and as soon as you mention cute fluffy animals it's all over the press.

STUART COLLEY

OutRage! came in for more flak when it challenged the Department of Health's ban on gay men donating blood, the implication being that because gay men, along with injecting drug users and other 'high-risk groups', might have infected blood, they should not be allowed to donate.

The blood transfusion campaign was basically a letter-writing campaign which was adopted by Peter and on the face of it seemed to be a very good idea, but as with a lot of these things it didn't seem to be thought out properly. There was an example that was given in an OutRage! press release that says a business man who goes on holiday to New York and has sex with a woman can come back and give blood yet is probably more at risk of HIV because he's had unprotected sex in New York than a gay man who's had protected sex in this country and has had safer sex all his life. Okay, you can see the dangers but given lack of resources in the blood transfusion service, the lack of an antigen test without a time lag on it, it just seemed completely pointless to be arguing lifting the blanket ban when the idea of a blanket ban is to protect not just heterosexual people but the whole country.

STUART COLLEY

Queer Intelligence Service

The OutRage! Queer Intelligence Service, effectively its Web page, began to produce in-your-face reports and articles designed to titillate and inform. In the summer of 1996, as attention turned to the military ban on homosexuality, OutRage! diverted its focus towards the Minister of Defence Michael Portillo, with a highly irreverent attack on him.

Deceitful and double dealing gossip concerning his 'gayness' are an insult to the queer community. Lame arguments put forward in support of these ridiculous rumours include:

1. Polly's a 'family values' MP, so where are the children?

2. The straight media makes constant insinuations (nevertheless too scared to say what they mean). They should know what they are on about.

Now who the fuck believes the breeder press?...

MICHAEL PORTILLO – THANK FUCK HE'S STRAIGHT.[3]

The campaign against Portillo became the focus of OutRage!'s presence at Pride on 6 July. Congregating at Parliament Square, they erected a 12-foot-high billboard with the words 'PORTILLO SCREWS QUEER SOLDIERS' in protest at his support for Section 28, an unequal age of consent, and the military ban on lesbians and gay men. Other placards included 'PORTILLO'S

BUGGERED THE ARMY', 'PORTILLO SUCKS' and 'PORTILLO: NO FRIEND OF DOROTHY'.

We were standing on the corner of Parliament with Big Ben and Parliament behind us and the whole of the Pride march went past. We had to hide the slogan with paper and plastic bags because we thought we'd be moved on before even getting there. Of the thousands and thousands of queers, everyone – except literally maybe one person – loved it. They stopped and cheered. Loads of people were rushing up and hugging us. It couldn't have gone better.

MARINA CRONIN

The Pride stunt was followed by an open letter to the Pride Trust expressing OutRage!'s concern at what it perceived as a commercialization of the event and loss of community and political focus. Following a tradition of discussing with Pride its direction and identity, OutRage! began by thanking the energy and commitment of Pride workers and volunteers, but then went on to make its own criticisms, including the fact that no banner stating it was 'Lesbian, Gay, Bisexual and Transgender Pride' was at the main stage and no mention was made of a continuing fight against anti-gay discrimination. OutRage! also criticized the fact that despite having a theme of 'Generations of Activism', only five GLF veterans were allowed two minutes on the main stage, and the main beneficiaries of Pride seemed to be straight-owned businesses. OutRage! went on to state:

We do not want Pride to become a dull and dour, politically correct event. We agree that it should have a Mardi Gras-style flavour. This does not, however, preclude also giving Pride a fun and energising political dimension. Pride must not become a mindless (if fabulous) once-a-year party where we pretend that we can dance away our second-class citizenship. We can't. On Clapham Common, we were 'slaves in a gilded cage'. We may have had a wild, brilliant Pride Festival, but that doesn't count for much when straight society fucks us over with impunity.[4]

OutRage! called for a broad-based specific human rights theme each year, a banner depicting the theme over the main stage and at the front of the march, stage time for activist and community groups, performers to say words of support for the theme, placards for marchers to carry and free stalls for non-profit community organizations.

In its letter, OutRage! also drew attention to the Home Office Minister Michael Howard's new proposals to crack down on sex offenders. This had been the theme of another of OutRage!'s cyber-offensives and letter-writing campaigns. Building on the campaign for a legal age of consent at 14,

OutRage! proposed that the 'Consultation Paper on Sentencing and Supervision of Sex Offenders' should follow the definition of a young person in the Indecency With Children Act 1960, that is that a child should be a young person under the age of 14. They went on to suggest that the requirement to register with the police currently being recommended by the consultation paper should exclude those convicted of consensual sex offences involving persons aged 14 or over and those convicted of similarly victimless offences where both partners are under 14 and of roughly comparable ages. In particular, OutRage! called for the largely gay and consensual offences of buggery, indecency, soliciting and homosexual acts on merchant ships to be deleted from the index of offences included in the terms of the Register.

A similar campaign was run by OutRage! to claim compensation for victims of aversion therapy. On 9 July, OutRage! called for an independent inquiry to uncover the truth about the extent and effects of aversion therapy, which involved the administration of electric shocks or nausea-inducing drugs coinciding with the patient being shown homoerotic images. In a letter to the Health Secretary Stephen Dorrell, OutRage! called for the establishment of an inquiry, compensation for those physically and psychologically affected, the establishment of specialized NHS counselling services to help gay and bisexual men sexually or emotionally damaged by aversion therapy and for the Department of Health to issue guidelines against the use of therapies that attempt to cure homosexuality. In addition, OutRage! wrote directly to the Royal College of Psychiatrists to officially renounce the practice of aversion therapy and apologize to the lesbian and gay community for its usage. The OutRage! campaign tied in with a BBC 2 documentary, *Sexual Aversion* broadcast on 8 August.

The campaigns against the blood transfusion ban on gay men, vivisection of animals, sentencing of offenders and aversion therapy constituted a move away from simple direct action – they represented interventions in political analysis and debate from a 'queer' perspective. OutRage! moved on with this formula with its campaign against Romania's anti-gay legislation in late 1996, calling for a boycott of their largest export, wine, resulting in a large-scale zap which stopped the Romanian National Opera's performance of *Aida* at the Royal Opera Hall on 20 October.

The end of 1996 saw OutRage! launching its most concerted and single-focused campaign since the 1992 'Equality Now' actions. 'Queer the Vote' was launched on 12 September, targeting the country's 30 most marginal constituencies for the forthcoming 1997 General Election with the aim of encouraging lesbians and gay men to register to vote before the closing date in mid-October. Where majorities were less than a hundred, and given that up to 10 per cent of the voting population were estimated by OutRage! to be lesbian or gay, the voting power of queer politics could have great effect. Recognizing that the General Election was also a time when lesbian and gay politics might leap forward in terms of debate and change, Stonewall launched a similar campaign. With OutRage! lobbying for people to register their votes, and Stonewall taking to the streets in Soho in order to give out publicity and queer postcards, the outside world might have been forgiven for thinking that the lesbian and gay community spoke with one voice – vote for change.

Death of an activist

OutRage! had always been the vision of a small number of people. One of those who attended the very first meeting was veteran GLF activist Martin Corbett. By 1996, it was clear that Martin was becoming increasingly unwell with progressing illnesses resulting from HIV infection. Even though he continued to help organize and demonstrate, the emotional and physical effort involved was beginning to take its toll.

Martin started to change in around September 1995. He was getting a lot more tired, and drinking as well. After the Christmas break he came back to OutRage!, and there was one meeting particularly where he came along and was really, really unwell. He had strange gestures and we were thinking what on earth are we going to do? Eventually he drove himself to St Mary's Hospital. I asked him why and he said he couldn't walk in a straight line anymore. Martin was so intelligent, so wonderful, such an important part of OutRage! I do actually feel that part of OutRage! getting a bit smaller and weaker was partly to do with Martin's input. He'd never have let the office get in such a mess, silly little things like that.

MARINA CRONIN

Martin stayed in hospital for a couple of weeks, and then went on to the London Lighthouse for care. Eventually, he went home and received 24 hour care. He died on 11 July 1996. In order to celebrate Martin's life, OutRage! arranged a 'queer political funeral' and candle-lit memorial procession on 10 August. While gay bar-goers and clubbers applauded, and straight football fans hurled bottles and shouted abuse, the procession made its way through the very heart of Soho to the London School of Economics, where the Gay Liberation Front had held its meetings. The event brought together representatives from nearly three decades of lesbian and gay activism. Martin Corbett's memorial service was itself a political event, paying homage to individual and collective acts of resistance.

We felt a march was in order because that was a pretty good symbol of what Martin was about. We had lots of friends and activists, and formed the march along the west end, including Compton's and St Martin's Lane, appropriately. It was lovely to have the OutRage! drum corps back. We did have some abuse, bottles thrown at us, from yobs in the West End. I felt, and others felt, that it was ironic that the worst of the abuse, the actual bottles being thrown, was on Old Compton Street, which was meant to be the street where everyone is free to be gay, it's our street. Well, of course, it's not our street. It's a London street. You can have as many cafes, bars as you like, it's still straight London. Then we marched from the Central Club where GLF videos and OutRage! videos were shown and went up to the LSE where GLF was born and the Sisters sang hymns and we laid flowers and candles. The candles were blowing out, quite a nice symbol of things going wrong – Martin hadn't organized it, so things went wrong.

MARINA CRONIN

Martin's funeral was in mid 1996 and already there were claims in the gay press that gay activism itself was dead. Indeed, by 1997, the sister activist group Lesbian Avengers had ceased activity, and fewer and fewer OutRage! actions or debates were being reported in either the gay or mainstream press. By 1997, OutRage! had lost its office in Peter Street. For at least seven years, OutRage! has been actively campaigning against homophobia, and with a new government in 1997 and three out gay members of Parliament elected, there is now hope for real change within Britain for lesbian and gay equality. Whether this does indeed mean there is no place for direct activism, or whether the clock will turn again, only time can tell. What is certain is that since its inception in 1990, OutRage! has been at the forefront of debates and interventions around sexuality and discrimination, and has had a significant cultural impact on not only lesbian and gay culture and politics, but also British culture and democracy in the very widest sense. Now was not like that then, indeed.

NOTES

1   OutRage! APPEAL FOR FUNDS, 1995.
2   OutRage! message to 'The March for the Animals', 20 June 1996.
3   OutRage! Queer Intelligence Service World Wide Web Page, 1996.
4   Open Letter To The Pride Trust, 18 July 1996.

AFTERWORD

Profit and Loss

As part of the interviews I carried out with current and former OutRage! members, one of the final questions I asked related to the more personal aspects of being involved in activism. It defined why they were involved, and why they left. Many people were involved for only a short time, either through frustration, anger, changes in personal circumstances or just plain old burn-out. For all of them, there were losses and benefits in their personal, political and financial lives. Inspiring, tiring, empowering, disillusioning, invigorating, heart-breaking and having fun were some of the conflicting emotions their involvement brought out. OutRage! was never just about the political – it was also about the process, and about group dynamics and loyalties. For most of the people who participated in the events chronicled in this book, things were never quite the same again.

It made me think more. It made me more aware of the world around me. It made me a more open person, because normally I don't do anything and I was the one that plodded around with all those leaflets. It made me talk to people more. I put a lot of effort in. I was always there in the office if placards needed doing. I went to all the pubs which I wouldn't have done.

BETH LANE

One of the benefits was being immensely empowered, that being gay was nothing to be ashamed of. Gay people had a voice. I was told to shut up, pretend you're straight, that's the best way to be gay. I realized it isn't. You know which friends were in OutRage! It also made me challenge my own beliefs about gay people, my own stereotypes. I met some really amazing people at OutRage!, some real role models. There were some real characters in OutRage! as well. I used to sit there and really fancy some people, other people I'd sit there in sheer amazement... The costs were mostly time for me.

KEVIN

When you first go along to a group like that, become empowered in that way, it's kind of going back to your teenage years, and you're going through puberty again. My voice broke at OutRage!, and my balls dropped!

DICE

I feel quite proud of it. I look back on it now and think we were having a huge amount of fun. I was also running around and having a huge amount of sex at the same time. I think the major benefit was some of the friendships I made. The costs were the degree of viciousness and unpleasantness that were involved in the group and the extent to which it blocked out the potential for me developing other areas of my life, for quite a long period. You become involved because you are looking for something and you may not even know that is what you're looking for. One of the things OutRage! really taught me was to be very wary of large groups of people and the energies they release because it can have a very insidious psychological effect. OutRage! was also very creative. It was a completely different way, from writing an article, of narrating a political idea and one which I found I was actually very good at. It developed my skills knowing how to manipulate the media, which I still use, but for completely different ends now!

KEITH ALCORN

It was a real antidote to Stonewall. It was a joy to watch something with that spirit. It does annoy me when people compare OutRage! to GLF, because they're such utterly different creatures. The problem for me was with people who claimed it was the true path, 'my organization is the only organization.'

LISA POWER

I often found myself after a meeting, at midnight, getting home and marking essays. I think I really encouraged Sarah to stay involved when perhaps she didn't want to. It was something we could do together. It did take up a lot of time, and I think our relationship suffered a bit because of it. My mother said, 'I don't know why you have to keep shouting about things all the time.' I opened my mind to things that I never would have thought about, I met people I'd never have met, I had conversations I'd never have had. I learned to use my body and my voice in a way which I hadn't done, which I think has fed into my acting and my comedy, my writing, my teaching even. It made me feel I belonged somewhere.

LYNNE SUTCLIFFE

The cost would be a temporary loss of sanity afterwards. I do still feel quite angry about that, and it's frustration with myself because I didn't achieve what I wanted to achieve. Nobody's allowed to fail. If you said you were going to do something, they assumed automatically you would do everything. If you came back to the next meeting with 'Oh, sorry, I forgot', there was a huge sigh of disappointment from the whole group and you'd sit there and crawl into a huge hole in the corner, saying 'I'm sorry, I'm sorry...' It's exhilarating and debilitating at the same time, like falling in love, the werdest range of emotions a person can go through. I can drop a few names – I met Derek Jarman briefly. If there was one thing I could ever change about OutRage!, it was the whistles, sitting in those meetings and tying those whistles and then having myself deafened at Pride. If I did it again, I probably wouldn't set up LABIA. I probably wouldn't take the minutes, because that stopped me putting my hands up because I'd have to stop writing. I hated it. I would try to be a better lesbian and turn up to more demos!

MEGAN RADCLIFFE

We spent so much time arguing. I've always been a big pragmatist and thought if someone's in the room, then try not to argue with them if basically you're coming from the same direction, allow them some leeway. There was so much hatred in the room. There was no back-slapping, haven't we done well. That's one of the unfortunate things of having a democracy, everybody has a say, regardless of what they're saying. One of the benefits was that things got out there. There were changes that were made and it improved my confidence in myself as a gay man. It's important if someone's giving you a hard time to say I don't think that's right. We were so unapologetic and so take us as you find us, I think that's great.

PATRICK McCANN

I've had my bicycle tyres slashed, bricks through my window, an arson attempt on my flat. I've been sent razor blades, dog shit, used condoms, and defaced newspaper photographs. At times it's felt like living through a civil war. It's left me feeling anxious and incredibly security conscious. I find it difficult to relax because there's this ever-present threat of what might happen. Three promising relationships broke up because of a combination of the huge workload that OutRage! has imposed upon me and because of the threats and assaults. One night I was having dinner in my flat with a new boyfriend and a brick came through the window, bounced across the table, smashing plates here, there and everywhere. He was totally traumatized by the experience and felt that he couldn't continue seeing me for the possibility of that kind of thing happening again. I found that very sad, but perhaps understandable.

These are some of the things that have been said… 'Tatchell should be castrated' (Sir Bernard Ingram, *Daily Express*), 'Homosexual terrorists' (*Daily Mail*), 'Public enemy no. 1' (*Sunday Times*), 'Prize Pervert' (*Daily Express*), 'Fascist' (*Daily Telegraph*), 'Pure poison' (*Evening Standard*), 'An enemy of the people' (*Daily Express*), 'The enemy within' (*Sunday Times*). Edwina Currie said I should be shot.

It's been tremendously uplifting and inspiring to be part of an organization which has made a tangible difference to the cultural perceptions of homosexuality, public awareness of anti-gay discrimination and self-help efforts of the queer community. By saying to society that we're no longer prepared to be kicked around, that's not only empowering for gay people in general, it's empowering for me too.

PETER TATCHELL

OutRage! gave gay people the opportunity to do things and show themselves, make a personal statement. People who weren't political came along. That for me was as important as the issues. It gave so many people the opportunity directly to participate, which maybe they don't need so much now.

ROB KEMP

If you ally yourself as an activist in England, you're always going to be seen as a crank. I don't think activism is cranky. Activism has costs, terrible costs. Actions become fetishized, become a complete identity. It gave me a real energy. I felt inadequate a lot of the time. I thought people looked to me for things that I wasn't always able to provide.

SIMON WATNEY

I can remember being accused by people of a similar political persuasion, on the left, who criticized me for being evangelical. It's too naïve to be like that. I was glad to go through that. The sad thing was, I came across a degree of personal hostility that shocked me. I'd been involved in the Labour Party for 13 years, and throughout the whole period of the most personal wrangling in the Labour Party, I've never come across the degree of personal nastiness that I came across in OutRage! That shocked me.

There's been no costs to me other than to open my eyes to the way that these people behaved.

STEVE STANNARD

I love the attention – media-attention-seeking whore-trollop, really. I don't know how much kudos there is associated with the group. There's probably no kudos at all anymore, if anything it's exactly the opposite, they see you as a bit sad. You're too involved, that you haven't got a life or something and there is a danger of doing that, getting involved too much, and you can lose yourself in it.

STUART COLLEY

In the space of the first three years of OutRage!, I'd lost three jobs on the trot because of politics; *Capital Gay* had sacked me, the *Pink Paper* had sacked me and *The Advocate* had sacked me. I became the most sacked gay journalist in history, and I actually quit print journalism and went into a different career. There was no separation between my political life, my work life and my social life. It was all gay politics, so if something went wrong in one area it just rippled into the others, and there was nothing to protect me. You can only last so long before you leave or go mad, or possibly both.

CHRIS WOODS

One of the things I remember was the passion involved. There was a lot of sex with other people, and on a personal level, it was one of the sexually most exciting times of my life. There was a great feeling of sexual possibility in the room, certainly for the men involved.

TOBY HOPKINS

All these things should be short-lived so that power groups can't form. It should be a bit anarchic, it should never have things that say 'This motion cannot be discussed for a year and a day.' It should be responding to whatever's going on at the time. If the Welfare State goes, we're in the shit, because so many battles have been won by lesbians and gays who are on the dole.

DAVE BUNNETT

Eventually I wondered to what extent it starts becoming an excuse for not doing much work in relation to yourself. I think, sometimes, looking at the heroism of activism, it's very easy to be a heroic activist, because you wake up every morning feeling like Napoleon Bonaparte, whereas it's perhaps more heroic, with a smaller 'h', to wake up and face the mundane, boring, drab, confusing tasks we have in life. I spent a year feeling utterly confused. For a year I was in freefall, I didn't know what the fuck I was doing, but I see it as recovery. For four years OutRage! was everything. I don't speak to my family, so it was the closest set of people I'd ever had. They were my social life. If it wasn't for OutRage!, I would have been back in Spain years ago.

FERNANDO GUASCH

It explains why I changed my role at my employer's, to commission lesbian and gay subjects within four months of joining OutRage! I thought what I was doing was part of OutRage!'s work, that it was direct action with a corporation with money. Having come out of OutRage!, I started to rapidly lose faith in gay politics and feel moments of severe alienation from gay people, a process of extreme bitterness and jadedness and feeling a lot of aggression to the gay world and gay people. Consequently, I lost enthusiasm for my books, and for my work. I felt post-Pride as a gay man, washed up politically and started to feel I was exacerbating the problem in the gay world with its fetishizing of consumer goods by producing these books. There was no politics involved in what I was doing with my work and so that lost me my motivation and I finished up resigning my job.

STEVE COOK

I left OutRage! not knowing who I was anymore. I hadn't realized how much of an identity it had given me. It really was who I was. We really felt it was us against the world, that we had a moral high ground which may or may not have been helpful. I remember Peter spoke at an SWP Marxism event, and I got up and spoke in favour of him, in favour of gay liberation politics, and then being denounced as 'radical posturing masking reactionary ideas'.

GRAHAM KNIGHT

My involvement with OutRage! taught me much too. Going back and researching its history enabled me to contact friends and people I later came to regard as friends. We connected immediately, and OutRage! taught me a way to relate to people, to look at what they do rather than what they say. I lost a certain amount of naïvety, and lost a lot of trust I would normally give to people. I no longer suffer fools gladly, and I don't have the same Good Gay Boy syndrome which was my traditional way of coping with homophobia. I'm much more ready to challenge assumptions, and patronizing liberals as well as out and out homophobes. And it's given me a long memory.

My own turning point was the age of consent debate, where we had won all the debates, and still lost the battle. It made me realize what cowards politicians are, and what a sham liberal democracy is. OutRage! empowered me, and encouraged me to challenge those people who set themselves up as authorities. Question, question, question.

Losses? There have been many – personal ones include those who have died, or friendships which have disappeared. There's also a sense of distance which remains from being involved in something as emotionally consuming as OutRage!, an inability to form friendships or partnerships unless motives are clear. There's a loss of hope, and faith in those who speak for us, who are supposed to work in my best interests as a gay man and as a citizen. Almost all of the the major institutions and personalities of the world in which I live have been targeted by OutRage!, proving that all of them have failed me and my kind at some time.

Yet despite this, I'm enormously proud and empowered because of my personal involvement with OutRage! I'd do it all again, and then some. I know when to smile, when to shout, and when to bite. There are signs that some of the measures we campaigned for are at last likely to become reality, which is fine. If and when equality arrives, I'll laugh, dance, weep and drink; in the morning, I'll wake up, smell the coffee and demand something better.

APPENDIX I

Chronology

1990

APRIL
30 Gay actor Michael Boothe is murdered in Ealing

MAY
1 OutRage!'s first meeting
31 Fundraising group formed – bank balance £16

JUNE
7 First demo at Hyde Park toilets against police entrapment
21 OutRage! votes to take over OLGA offices at the London Lesbian and Gay Centre
30 Action against Revolutionary Communist Party stall at Pride
Laying of wreath at Cenotaph

JULY
10 March with Ealing Lesbian and Gay Forum at protest of murder of gay actor Michael Boothe
12 Demo by Brighton activists at Princess Diana's speech at the International Congress of the Family, Brighton
17 OutRage! demo against International Congress of the Family
19 OutRage! vote to buy whistles for fundraising
27 First OutRage! Whistle Patrol

AUGUST
16 Demo outside Scotland Yard
30 Zap on Paradise Club, Islington

SEPTEMBER
5 Kiss-In at Piccadilly Circus
10 OutRage! outreach trip to Manchester
22 OutRage! supports Black Lesbian and Gay Group picket of Brixton Police Station
OutRage! delivers first protest letter to Brief Encounter over their ban on same-sex kissing
28 Leafletting of Brief Encounter
30 Meeting to discuss Policing Initiative

OCTOBER
1 Support ACT UP demo at Texaco HQ
2 First Policing Initiative meeting with the Metropolitan Police
4 Steve Stannard ousted as treasurer – discussion of sectarian interests within OutRage!
10 Kiss-In at Brief Encounter
19 Demo against Ealing MP Harry Greenway

NOVEMBER
5 OutRage! supports Gay Rights In Prison demo at Wandsworth Prison
27 Market Tavern benefit for OutRage!, hosted by Jeremy Joseph

DECEMBER
3 March from Coleherne to Earls Court Police Station
9 Winter Pride – March, OutRage! panto, headshaving and merchandise stall
17 OutRage! Christmas Celebration for London's Extended Family, Covent Garden
20 OutRage! sets up the Coalition for Lesbian and Gay Rights

1991

JANUARY
10 Queer Nation cell structure adopted by OutRage!
13 Initial meeting of the Coalition for Lesbian and Gay Rights
14 Scrubbing Parliament Clean of Homophobia

FEBRUARY
3 Screening of *The Garden* benefit for OutRage! at the Electric Cinema
6 Mass Turn-in of OutRage! 'Sex Criminals' at Bow Street
14 Washing Union Jack Clean of Homophobia – ILGA international actions
16 Lesbian and Gay Rights Coalition National March and Benefit at Paradise
21 Zap on Paradise Club over alleged mistreatment of two lesbians

MARCH
11 Filming of *Edward II*; spontaneous zap against Cliff Richard
17 Public meeting at the London Lesbian and Gay Centre on use of the word 'queer'

23 Zap on Annual General Meeting of National Viewers' and Listeners' Association
29 Zap at Home Office against Paragraph 16

APRIL
4 Affinity groups adopted
13 Liberation mass demo in Manchester
19 Zap against Archbishop of Canterbury, George Carey and burning of 'queer martyrs'
21 Whores of Babylon Zap of Rev Lister's church in Tufnell Park over his homophobic newsletter

MAY
16 Renaming of Office Group to Queer Accountants Never Go Out (QUANGO)
21 Zap on Isle of Man stall at Shipping Exhibition, Barbican
23 Perverts Undermining State Scrutiny (PUSSY) set up

JUNE
12 Queer Wedding at Nelson's Column, Trafalgar Square
13 OutRage! South Kiss-In, Southampton Town Centre
21 OutRage! Whistle Patrol and midnight performance of TeaTrolley on Clapham Common
27 Alan Shea from the Isle of Man attends an OutRage! meeting

JULY
5 Opening of Tinwald, Isle of Man
9 Zap on Brief Encounter over their 'Bring A Fish' poster
18 OutRage! Family Group picket of DSS HQ against the Family Support Bill
31 Faggots Rooting Out Closeted Sexuality (FROCS) Press Conference

AUGUST
1 Queer Reality #1 produced
7 Exorcism of Lambeth Palace
16 OutRage! merchandise and safer-sex stall on Hampstead Heath
17 Work It Girl (WIG) action in Oxford Street
21 Queer Heritage zap at Epsom cruising ground
22 Launch of Focus Groups
23 Big Nancy cabaret benefit for OutRage!
26 OutRage! wins Vauxhall Tavern Sports Day
27 Queers Underground Asserting the Right to Ride Every Line Safely (QUARRELS) Tube action
30 Queer Planet zap against Amnesty International
31 OutRage! supports Gay Rights In Prison demo at Pentonville Prison

SEPTEMBER
1 Queer Heritage zap at Hampstead men and women's bathing ponds

13 Socialist Lesbians And Gays (SLAGS) action against The Guardian newspaper with OutRage! OutRage! stall on Hampstead Heath
14 Condom clear-up of Hampstead Heath
23 OutRage! boycott of the Guardian
25 Lesbians Answer Back In Anger (LABIA) first meeting

OCTOBER
5 Hampstead Heath litter cruise
9 Queer Heritage demo at Epsom Crown Court
31 First demo at State Opening of Parliament

NOVEMBER
7 LABIA Jennifer Saunders action
17 First zap against Living Waters ex-gay movement at St Michael's Church, Belgravia
24 Open meeting on future of Coalition for Lesbian and Gay Rights
27 SISSY action at Haverstock School, Kentish Town

DECEMBER
1 Zap at St Michael's Church, Belgravia – 11 arrested
3 Zap at Church of England press release regarding homosexuality
6 OutRage! attends demo against French right-winger Jean-Marie Le Pen at Charing Cross Hotel
12 Ivan Thoms, South African gay campaigner, attends OutRage! meeting

1992

JANUARY
26 Demo outside Evening Standard Awards Ceremony

FEBRUARY
6 Equality Now March on Parliament – 45 arrests
15 Demo against Benetton shops over advertising campaign
20 Equality Now 'Queering' of military statues and demo at Ministry of Defence

MARCH
5 Equality Now Wink-In at Piccadilly Circus
19 Equality Now application to register lesbian and gay partnerships
First zap against Conservative Family Protection Group

APRIL
2 Equality Now Employment demos:
Fat Arrowsmith hands in letter to Department of Employment
Demo in support of Alison Halford at New Scotland Yard
Demo outside High Court at Jason Donovan/The Face libel trial

10 OutRage! demo outside 10 Downing Street – three arrested
11 Stickering zap against Guns 'N' Roses records, Tower Records, Piccadilly Circus
16 Equality Now Teenage Turn-In and 'Bend Over For Your Member' demo outside Parliament
18 Stickering zap against Guns 'N' Roses, Virgin Megastore
25 LABIA attempt to set up a Lesbian cruising ground on Hampstead Heath
30 Equality Now zap on Tory HQ against anniversary of Section 28; free sample of homosexuality

MAY
6 Demo at State Opening of Parliament
8 OutRage! demonstrates against the film *Basic Instinct*
18 Double zap against Clerical and Medical at their Bristol HQ and registered offices in London
29 'Safer Cruising' action on Clapham Common

JUNE
25 Abolition of focus groups

JULY
8 Demo against military queerbashing at Earls Court Royal Tournament
25 End of Equality Now – March on Downing Street

AUGUST
4 Invasion of Vatican Embassy
8 OutRage! British National Party watch in Soho
9 Disruption of service at Westminster Cathedral

SEPTEMBER
20 Attempted crucifixion at Westminster Cathedral
21 Zap against Supt Hames, Obscene Publications Squad, at National Women's Council Meeting

OCTOBER
9 Hyde Park 'Cruise-In'
27 OutRage! attend launch of *Daring To Speak Love's Name*, Westminster Central Hall
31 Coalition for Lesbian and Gay Rights March

NOVEMBER
9 Demo at Royal Mail HQ in support of worker Steven Watts
30 Zap on London Rubber Company HQ for World AIDS Day

DECEMBER
1 World AIDS Day demo at Downing Street with ACT UP
7 Demo at Royal Mail HQ in Cambridge
8 Demo against Buju Banton outside Hammersmith Palais
10 Storming of Royal Mail HQ in Cambridge

1993

JANUARY
17 Raid on South Oxley Community Church used to 'cure' homosexuality

FEBRUARY
13 Queer Carnival, Soho

MARCH
26 OutRage! 'Spank-In' protest against Spanner Appeal
Protest at BBC against Shabba Ranks's appearance on Top of the Pops
Action at Harrow School
28 OutRage! due to be evicted from London Lesbian and Gay Centre

APRIL
4 Zap on Cardinal Basil Hume, Palm Day procession, Westminster Cathedral
15 Phone zap on *Crimewatch*
22 Invasion of BBC building
26 Protest against John Birt, Royal Television Society meeting, Whitehall

MAY
22 OutRage! moves into new offices at 5 Peter Street, Soho
26 Zap on John Major's old school, Rutlish, in Wimbledon

JUNE
3 OutRage! starts meeting at Covent Garden Community Centre

JULY
1 OutRage! disrupts Haringey Council meeting after dismissal of David Morgan
22 Zap against Crown Prosecution Service

AUGUST
26 Third Birthday Party and Relaunch

SEPTEMBER
OutRage! quits London Lesbian and Gay Policing Initiative
13 OutRage! and ACT UP zap Bromley Council meeting
16 Zap at Western Marble Arch Synagogue in protest at comments made by Rabbi Jakobovits
22 Zap with ACT UP against Benetton HQ

OCTOBER
16 OutRage! attends ANL/ARA march against fascism in Plumstead

NOVEMBER
12 Peter Tatchell confronts PM John Major
18 Demo at State Opening of Parliament

30 Demo with Welsh group Dicclon against Rabbi Jakobovits at St David's Hall, Cardiff

DECEMBER
1 Distribution of condoms and safer-sex resources outside Christ the King Sixth Form College, Lewisham
18 Urban Glamour Assault

1994

FEBRUARY
19 Derek Jarman dies
21 Candle-light vigil, age of consent vote, Parliament. Age of consent lowered from 21 to 18
23 OutRage! members confront John Major as he opens intensive care unit at King's College Hospital

MARCH
14 Age of Dissent March on Parliament

APRIL
7 Demo outside the Danish Embassy, asking Danes to invade Britain
16 OutRage! Mersey demo against MP Bob Parry for voting against an equal age of consent
Zap on Labour's National executive meeting

MAY
7 Teenage Turn-In, Charing Cross Police Station
29 Zap on Cardinal Basil Hume's blessing of the new Catechism, Westminster Cathedral

JUNE
5 Demo against Benetton at *Quilts of Love* exhibition, Hyde Park

JULY
10 Zap at Hampstead Heath bathing pond
26 OutRage! joins march against Criminal Justice Bill, Trafalgar Square
Inaugural Lesbian Avengers meeting

AUGUST
7 Queers Against Fundamentalism demo against Wembley Muslim Fundamentalist rally, subsequently adopted as an OutRage! action
19 Zap against Sgt Paul Canneaux, Heath warden responsible for policing Hampstead Heath

SEPTEMBER
5 Handing out cruising leaflets at Battersea Park
24 Zap against the Courage Trust's Open Day at Chorleywood

OCTOBER
9 OutRage! attends march against the Criminal Justice Bill

22 Zap of Bishop Michael Turnbull at his enthronement in Durham

NOVEMBER
15 Zap of Synod Press Conference and confrontation of Bishop of Durham at Greenwich University Awards Ceremony
16 OutRage! zaps on State Opening of Parliament
18 OutRage! National Tour starts
27 Zap at Westminster Cathedral, helium-filled condoms released
30 'Outing' of ten Church of England bishops at General Synod

DECEMBER
18 OutRage! disrupts enthronement of John Gladwin as Bishop of Guildford

1995

JANUARY
10 Letter written to 20 gay MPs urging them to come out

FEBRUARY
21 Candle-light vigil, anniversary of age of consent vote

MARCH
20 MP James Kilfedder dies – OutRage! blamed by the press

JULY
21 Zap of True Freedom Trust Turnabout meeting, Westbourne Park Baptist Church
22 OutRage! disrupts farewell service for Bishop of St Albans

AUGUST
13 Protest against Assembly for Islam, Trafalgar Square
18 Demonstration against President Mugabe, Zimbabwe High Commission
23 Zap of Living Waters International Conference at St Michael's, Belgravia

SEPTEMBER
8 Queer Jihad against Al-Muhajiroun at Speaker's Corner, Hyde Park

OCTOBER
1 OutRage! and Lesbian Avengers picket Sainsbury's over funding anti-gay religious movements

NOVEMBER
12 Laying of wreath at Cenotaph for Queer Remembrance Day
27 OutRage! nail list of queer demands to Westminster Abbey door

OutRage! join GLF 25th Anniversary, Highbury Fields

DECEMBER
19 OutRage! zaps Queen's annual Royal Christmas Staff Ball

1996

FEBRUARY
13 OutRage! launch campaign for equal age of consent at 14 outside House of Commons
21 OutRage! join NUS for 'Stamp Out Homophobia' rally, House of Commons

MARCH
2 Zap at Fulham Police Station – daubing of Queers Bash Back

JUNE
20 OutRage! message of support read out by Chrissie Hynde at 'The March for Animals' Washington, DC

JULY
2 OutRage! comment on Home Office consultation paper on sex offenders
6 OutRage! billboard – 'Portillo Screws Queer Soldiers' in Parliament Square during Lesbian, Gay, Bisexual and Transgender Pride March
9 OutRage! launch campaign for compensation for victims of aversion therapy

AUGUST
10 Queer Political Funeral of Martin Corbett and march through Soho

SEPTEMBER
12 OutRage! launches 'Queer the Vote' campaign

OCTOBER
20 OutRage! zaps Romanian National Opera at Royal Albert Hall

APPENDIX 2

The Philosophy of OutRage! An Interview with Peter Tatchell

London, February 1997

Ian Lucas One of OutRage!'s founders, Simon Watney, is credited with saying that OutRage! was like a machine, into which you put homosexuals and get out lesbians and gay men. Many of the people I interviewed saw OutRage! as a process, a form of group therapy. Is that a view you would share?

Peter Tatchell OutRage! doesn't have an agenda about changing the people who get involved. It's about providing the space for queers to change themselves. One of the many great strengths of OutRage! is its grass-roots democracy. Unlike Stonewall, which is a self-selected organization which no ordinary lesbian or gay person can join, OutRage! is totally open and accessible. To get involved, you don't have to sign a membership form or pay a subscription. All you have to do is turn up at the weekly meetings. That gives you the right to speak, vote, in the determination of policy. There's no ideological test that people have to go through, other than a commitment to fight for the self-determination and human rights of queers. Our openness means that we are by far the most accountable group within the lesbian and gay community. If anybody doesn't agree with what we're doing, they've got the right to come to a meeting and say so, and they've got a right to seek to overturn our policy. No other organization has that level of openness and accessibility.

OutRage! has always relied on donations from the public to achieve its aims. How has it continued with such tight financial resources?

OutRage! has been incredibly successful, particularly given its small size and lack of funds. On average, an annual budget for OutRage! has been about £6000. That covers the office, telephones, press liaison. It's incredible value for money. Everyone in OutRage! is a volunteer. Often, we don't even get expenses. Many times we pay for things out of our own pocket. Stonewall has an annual budget of over £400,000 a year, several full-time paid staff, a whole range of office facilities and campaign resources that we just don't have. Some journalists have often commented that OutRage!'s profile and effectiveness is comparable to that of an organization like Greenpeace. Greenpeace has an annual budget of £2.5 million and over 60 full-time paid staff. For us to be able to have such an impact given our lack of paid staff and proper campaign resources is an amazing achievement.

Do you see advantages in the organization not having paid workers?

We've always felt that the voluntary principle is important. Our motivation is idealism, not careerism. Although it's impossible to run a group without an element of differentiation between the members, it's important the differentiation is based on skills and commitment rather than an imposed hierarchical structure. We've never had any officers or leaders such as a chair or a director. It's always infuriated me personally and everyone else in OutRage! that the press often describe me as a leader of OutRage! I'm not, I don't want to be. I'm no more important than anybody else in the group. I do have particular adeptness in handling the media, but just because I'm often the spokesperson for the group, that doesn't make me more important than anyone else. Contrary to the way it's often portrayed, my view doesn't always hold sway in OutRage! I've been outvoted on many, many, many issues. In retrospect, sometimes that's been a good thing.

You say that you are not the leader of OutRage!, but you often do much of the media work. I know that you crafted many of the press releases issued by OutRage!, for example.

Often I've been asked to draft press releases on behalf of OutRage because I'm a journalist by profession and I've got the expertise and know how to do that job. Mostly I've always made sure that other people are included on the press release. I've tried to include everyone within the core activist group as a spokesperson on a more or less rotating basis. There's also an attempt at gender parity wherever possible, so that a press release will often contain a quote from both a lesbian and a gay man in OutRage!

We've always attempted to be a democratic, egalitarian, non-hierarchical, grass-roots organization. In that context, singling one person out is counter to the ethos of the group. One of the reasons that has happened is partly because prior to the establishment of OutRage!, I was well known to the media, largely because I stood as a Labour candidate for the Bermondsey by-election and to a lesser extent because of my subsequent writing and activism on gay issues. Even before the establishment of OutRage! everyone in the media knew my name and telephone number

One of the problems was that many people in OutRage! had full-time jobs or studies so they weren't available. By and large the media works on a nine-to-five schedule. Because I'm freelance and work from home, I was available. On a lot of lesbian and gay rights issues, I've done ground-breaking research and investigative journalism, so I have a huge compendium of facts and knowledge at my fingertips. When the media need information, often when they've gone to other people in OutRage!, they haven't got it so they end up coming back to me.

Having said that the media use you for information, much media attention on you personally has been disparaging and critical.

My name has been both a strength and a weakness. On the one hand it's given the media a readily accessible and knowledgeable contact for the group, but it's also meant that my profile has superseded that of other members. I've always had the view that the media is something to be treated with suspicion and caution, given its homophobic record, but it's also something which can be used beneficially to promote awareness and understanding of lesbian and gay issues. It's a very dicey game – sometimes you win, sometimes you lose. If OutRage! had adopted a paranoid attitude towards the media, as some other lesbian and gay groups had done, we never would have been so successful in raising public consciousness about key aspects of homophobic discrimination. Sometimes we got our fingers burnt, but overall, on balance, the effect has been very positive.

OutRage! has defined itself as a 'direct action' group, but I've noticed, especially recently, that much of its work has been along more traditional lines – articles, information, letter-writing campaigns. Do you see this as direct action?

OutRage! has survived three times as long as the Gay Liberation Front. We are the oldest, longest-established lesbian and gay direct action group in the world. One of the reasons for our longevity is our flexibility and adaptability. We haven't dogmatically stuck to direct action to the exclusion of everything else. All through OutRage!'s history, direct action has been the core, but there have always been elements of advice, support and counselling, the fighting of individual cases, and a very strong element of letter-writing and negotiating with the authorities as a follow-up to direct action. I'd liken OutRage!'s direct action strategy to a form of non-violent guerrilla war. We're a small organization confronting immensely powerful homophobic individuals and institutions. We cannot hope to defeat them in a full-frontal assault. What we *can* do, through a war of attrition, is harass and wear down the supporters of homophobia and the institutions that sustain discrimination.

OutRage! is constantly challenging homophobia. We're calling the people who perpetuate discrimination to account. Often we confront them personally face to face in a bid to shame, ridicule and embarrass them, to destroy their credibility and to make them rethink whether being homophobic is worth all the difficulties we could cause them. It's very rare that we win a set-piece battle, but the long-term effect of ceaselessly challenging homophobia is to wear down and undermine our enemies.

There have often been tensions between OutRage! as a direct action group and Stonewall as a lobbying organization. Do you see the two forms of campaigning as incompatible with each other?

OutRage! partly came into existence to fill a gap created by all the things Stonewall wasn't. OutRage! had an agenda beyond equality. While we accept that equality is an important principle, we also acknowledge that it has its limitations. Equal rights within straight society inevitably means equality on heterosexual terms. We conform to their agenda. OutRage! has always sought to articulate a post-equality agenda which seeks to renegotiate the values, institutions and laws of straight culture, challenging not just homophobia but the authoritarian and puritanical nature of social institutions. What we want is a new agenda which will not only safeguard the human and sexual rights of lesbians, gays and bisexuals but ultimately do likewise for straight people as well. Our agenda is about transforming society, not conforming to it. Stonewall has always had an assimilationist agenda, it doesn't question the parameters of heterosexual society.

Most people in OutRage! have always accepted that there is a role for different tactics. Sometimes direct action is the number one priority. At other times negotiation might be important. Lobbying and direct action need not be mutually exclusive. They can often complement each other. We have frequently found that OutRage! direct action has pushed lesbian and gay issues into the headlines, promoting public awareness and debate which has then put homophobes under pressure and enabled more orthodox lobbying groups like Stonewall to be invited to the negotiating table. Although we have different tactics and aims from Stonewall, OutRage! has always tried to work with them and sought to acknowledge their role and contribution. That generosity has often not been reciprocated. Stonewall frequently comes across as attempting to claim the credit for everything that's ever been achieved in the community. They tend not to acknowledge other groups, not just OutRage! but the Lesbian and Gay Christian Movement, GALOP, Lesbian and Gay Employment Rights and many others. Stonewall styles itself as *the* Lesbian and Gay lobbying group, not *a* lesbian and gay lobbying group but *the* lesbian and gay lobbying group. That smacks of arrogance and empire building. It has a whiff of an attempt to monopolize the whole agenda for themselves.

One of the criticisms levelled at direct action groups such as OutRage! is that you are just creating stunts, amateur dramatics. Is OutRage! just a group of publicity seekers?

The people who criticize OutRage!'s actions as mere stunts are by and large living in the past. They are wedded to an old-style leftist idea that the way to protest is by organizing a march and a rally. That has been done to death, it's become predictable, routine, boring and un-newsworthy unless of course you get half a million people. OutRage! has had the sense to recognize that we live in a modern telecommunications era where the main means of social communication is through newspapers, television and radio. A march through a major city can reach maybe a few thousand people who might happen to witness it passing, but a creative exciting direct action stunt can generate news and current affairs coverage that will result in the issues getting out to a wider audience of millions. The OutRage! agenda is about promoting public awareness and debate concerning homophobic discrimination, generating discussions. The most effective way to achieve that is to do something that gets the issue reported.

None of us in OutRage! is interested in getting publicity for ourselves. Many times we've been approached by newspapers and television programme makers for personal profiles about people within the group, but every time we've turned down those proposals. We're not interested in speaking to the media except to articulate the ideas and issues that OutRage! is fighting for. If I was interested in personal publicity I would have accepted some of the suggested offers that I take up a career in television. Over the years it's been suggested to me several times that I apply for certain jobs presenting television programmes or doing research and news reporting. The BBC wanted to do a major television programme, possibly a series, on the people behind OutRage! but we turned it down because we felt it would focus on personalities to the exclusion of the lesbian and gay equality agenda. Over the years OutRage! has fed hundreds and hundreds of stories to TV and radio programme makers and the media and often we haven't featured in those ourselves, but we've got coverage for couples seeking to adopt children or people facing discrimination in employment and so on.

Even negative publicity isn't always as bad as it seems. There may be some short-term damage but the longer-term effect is to help normalize homosexuality. In a society that wants to keep homosexuality invisible, anything that can help create visibility has a beneficial long-term effect. A lot of the fears and phobias around gay sexuality arise because people are scared of the unknown or things which they regard as unusual or odd. Over time it becomes normalized and that is part of the process of undermining people's fears and anxieties.

In 1992, when the focus groups were abolished, OutRage! was accused of being a white, male, middle-class club, that it didn't represent the views of other groups within the queer community. Do you accept that criticism?

The caucus groups had become monopolized by people who were hostile to the aims and objectives of OutRage! Their first loyalty was not to fighting homophobia but to other political agendas, even to other political groups. They were coming to OutRage! on behalf of revolutionary socialist sects in a bid to take over the group. Most of the women in OutRage! were not involved in LABIA. Most of the working-class people did not participate in the working-class caucus. Most of the black people in OutRage! were not in ETHNIC. When the vote to disband the caucus groups was taken, there were about 60 people at the meeting. From my recollection only three people voted against disbanding the groups. None of the women in the meeting voted in favour of retaining LABIA, none of the black people wanted to retain the black group.

OutRage! doesn't have the same profile it did a few years ago. Do you think, given the current political climate, that as an organization it has a future?

Every organization has its birth, life and death. No group goes on forever – just think of the Whigs and Independent Labour Party, now consigned to history. There may well come a time when OutRage! is no longer necessary or justified, but that time is not yet. Over recent months and years OutRage! is still doing direct action and is still setting the agenda of lesbian and gay civil rights.

Index

ACT UP (AIDS Coalition To Unleash Power) 6–8, 21, 63, 122, 143, 162, 164
age of consent 9, 28, 169, 171–5, 180, 182, 187 190, 201, 202, 214, 217, 218, 228
Ahmed, Aamir 72, 77, 85, 89, 95, 96, 98, 123, 143, 150, 176
AIDS 1, 8, 10, 25–6, 31, 85, 122, 143, 145, 148, 154, 162, 166, 168, 192, 215, 216, 217, 220
AIDS Coalition To Unleash Power, see ACT UP
Ajay 24, 44, 51, 95, 123, 124, 129
Alcorn, Keith 7, 8, 13, 14, 15, 16, 17, 18, 20, 22, 23 26, 28, 33, 43, 44, 45, 46, 52 53, 130, 224
Allison, David 8, 21, 22, 27, 151
Al-Mass'ari, Dr Muhammad 211
Al-Muhajiroun 210, 211
Amnesty International 91–2
Anderton, James 7
Archer, Rob 141
Arnold, David 10, 107, 111, 118, 119, 124, 127, 128, 137, 139
Arrowsmith, Pat 112

Baker, Kenneth (MP) 60–1, 80
Bakewell, Joan 188
Banton, Buju 144–5
Basic Instinct 144
BBC (British Broadcasting Corporation) 5, 145–8
Beeson, John 3, 7–8, 21, 33, 105, 115, 117, 138, 150
Belfast Telegraph 199, 200
Bellos, Linda 116

Benetton 8, 122, 162–6
Blair, Tony (MP) 178
Blunkett, David (MP) 177, 178
Boffin, Tessa 37
Booth, Hartley (MP) 205
Boothe, Michael 14, 19
Brief Encounter 35–7, 93
British Broadcasting Corporation, see BBC
Broomhall, Shane 17, 26, 27, 43, 44, 64, 65, 66, 67, 68, 69, 70, 71, 75, 76, 89, 181
Brown, Gordon (MP) 178
Brown, Michael (MP) 198
Bunnett, David 23, 28, 31, 32, 42, 45, 46, 84, 85, 221
Burgess, Mike 22
Butler, Chris (MP) 49

Campaign for Homosexual Equality (CHE) 3–5, 16
Capital Gay 3, 15, 22, 39, 45, 55, 161, 201, 227
Carey, George (Archbishop of Canterbury) 74–5, 195
Cashman, Michael 9, 181
Cave, Nick 79, 100, 103, 104, 106, 107, 127, 137, 156, 157, 173
Central Station 124
CHE, see Campaign for Homosexual Equality
Children's Society 193, 206
Clarke, Margi 137
Clerical Medical Investment 125–6
Cole, Michael 82
Colley, Stuart 172, 173, 183, 192–3, 202, 203, 204, 206, 211, 213, 214, 215, 216, 217, 227
Combat 18 200
Compton's 124, 221

Cook, Steve 103, 105, 116, 117, 118, 123, 124, 127, 128, 130, 131, 133, 135, 138, 146, 147, 149, 151, 160, 162, 163, 164, 165, 166, 176, 178, 182, 183, 188, 190, 228
Corbett, Martin 16, 21, 27, 40, 108, 110, 124, 150, 164, 174, 176, 203, 204, 213, 220–1
Corbyn, Jeremy (MP) 105
Courage Trust 187, 193, 204–5
Crimewatch 146–7
Criminal Justice Bill 1991 49–51, 54
Croll, Ben 162, 163, 164
Cronin, Marina 179, 200, 202, 203, 204, 205, 206, 210, 212, 213, 214, 218, 220, 221
Crown Prosecution Service 156–7, 164
Currie, Edwina (MP) 171, 173, 215, 226

DAFT (Dykes And Faggots Together) 4
Daily Mail 67, 174, 226
Daily Telegraph 200, 226
Dalziel, William 13
Daring to Speak Love's Name 139–40
de Marco, Nick 118, 126, 127, 128, 129, 176
Derbyshire, Philip 39
Diana, Princess of Wales 27
Dice 113, 115, 123, 134, 138, 146, 149, 150, 153, 154, 162, 164, 165, 168, 177, 178, 179, 188, 192, 193, 203, 204, 224
Donovan, Jason 64–5, 113
Dorrell, Stephen (MP) 219
Douglas, Michael 144
Durant, Sir Anthony 171

242 | Index

Dykes And Faggots Together, *see* DAFT

Ealing Lesbian and Gay Forum 26–7
Edge, Simon 51, 57, 70, 186, 199, 201
The Edge 150
Edward II 59–60
Elizabeth II, Queen 93–4, 116, 187, 213
Epsom and Ewell Herald 83
Equality Now campaign 100, 101–19, 121, 219
ETHNIC (Expanding The Non-Indigenous Contingent) 94
Evening Standard 84, 121–2, 153, 226
exorcism of Lambeth Palace 75–7

The Face 65, 113
Fairbrass, Richard 115
'Family Christmas' (Covent Garden) 46–7, 49
Fitzpatrick, Dr Michael 25
Fong, Regina 47, 54
Foster, Jodie 63
Frazer, Jean 16, 43
French, Matthew 66
Friend helpline 38
FROCS (Faggots Rooting Out Closeted Sexuality) 63–71, 189

GALOP (Gay London Policing Group)
GALZ (Gays And Lesbians of Zimbabwe) 211, 212
Gambaccini, Paul 67
Gaultier, Jean-Paul 18
Gay Activists Alliance 4
Gay Business Association 38, 39
Gay Liberation Front, *see* GLF
Gay Men Fighting AIDS, *see* GMFA
Gay News 2
Gay's the Word 23, 40, 88
Geffen, David 143
Gibson, Mel 63
Girvin, Martin 76, 78, 79
Gladwin, John (Bishop of Guildford) 193

GLF (Gay Liberation Front) 2–3, 4, 16, 21, 27, 33, 40, 53, 206, 218, 220, 221, 224
GMFA (Gay Men Fighting AIDS) 26, 83, 210
Gorman, Theresa (MP) 62
Grace, Della (Del) 87, 88
Graham, Sarah 147, 148
Green, Sue 164, 165
Greenaway, Harry (MP) 27
Greenhalgh, Hugh 171
Guasch, Fernando 47, 79, 103, 109, 112, 116, 117, 118, 125, 131, 136, 139, 140, 148, 150, 155, 160, 161, 162, 163, 165, 166, 168, 177, 178, 182, 183, 187, 188, 190, 193, 195, 201, 227–8
Guinness, Rev. Christopher 77, 78, 79
Gulf War 52
Guns 'N' Roses 143–4

Halsbury, Lord 5
Hames, Supt Michael 138–9
Hamilton, Angus 55, 164
Haringey Council 153–4
Harrington, Martin 74, 78, 83, 84, 85, 92, 98, 123, 128, 135, 150
Hegley, John 54
Hews, Sarah 110
Hizb-ur-Tahrir 184, 210
Homo Promos 82
Hope, David (Bishop of London) 194, 195
Hopkins, Roz 180
Hopkins, Toby 6, 20, 21, 23, 24, 27, 28, 46, 62, 74, 75, 81, 227
Houston, Whitney 63
Howard, Michael (MP) 218
Howes, Julian 213
Human Embryology and Fertilization Bill 19, 28
Hume, Cardinal Basil 132, 137, 138, 185
Hurlbert, David, 11, 14, 17, 19, 22, 43, 61, 66, 68, 74, 75
Hynde, Chrissie 216

Icebreakers 3
Independent 34, 67, 194
'In-Rage' 58

International Conference for the Family 27–9
Ireland, Colin 154–5
Irie, Tippa 145
Iris Trust 9
Irskine, Ian 13
Isle Of Man 80–2, 138, 139

Jackson, John 3, 28, 33, 97, 98, 99, 109, 126, 144, 151, 160, 177, 191, 192, 198, 204
Jakobovits, Lord (Chief Rabbi) 131, 159–61
Jarman, Alan 53, 89, 99, 100, 128, 174
Jarman, Derek 52, 58–60, 67, 85, 104, 109, 121, 151, 172, 174, 225
Jeanes, Adam 8, 21, 22, 27, 32, 35, 42, 45
Jewish Chronicle 160, 161
Jones, Phil 174, 187, 188, 189, 191, 193–4, 198, 200, 201, 215
Joseph, Jeremy 37, 47, 174
Justice for Women 97

Kemp, Rob 55, 92, 144, 147, 151, 172, 173, 174, 176, 226
Kevin 117, 176, 223–4
Kierney, James 24, 37, 82, 84, 89, 90, 96, 115, 123, 124, 126, 150
Kilfedder, James (MP) 199–201
King, Edward 8, 25, 34, 166
King, Tom (MP) 107
Kirby, David 122
Kiss-In 31–4, 101, 108
Knight, Graham 60, 61, 74, 76, 77, 95, 102, 109, 115, 117, 118, 127, 129, 130, 145, 146, 147, 149, 162, 177, 228
Kramer, Larry 7

LABIA (Lesbians Answer Back In Anger) 94, 96–7, 122, 128, 225
Labour Party 177–9, 226
Ladies' Excuse Me 94
Lane, Beth 52, 59, 61, 81, 82, 90, 106, 107, 149, 168, 177, 178, 223

Lesbian and Gay Campaign Against Racism and Fascism, *see* LGCARF
Lesbian and Gay Rights Coalition 35, 50–5
Lesbian Avengers 180–1, 192, 205, 206, 210, 211, 221
Lesbians and Gays Support the Miners 42
Let's Rap 144
LGCARF (Lesbian and Gay Campaign Against Racism and Fascism) 54, 126–31, 176
Liberty 67, 187
Lind, Stephen 105
LINK 94, 95
Living Waters 77–80, 148–9, 205
Livingstone, Ken (MP) 54
Local Government Act 1988 ('Section 28') 1, 5–6, 51, 97, 115–16, 198, 217
Lofty 62, 65, 66, 67, 69, 170, 189
London Lesbian and Gay Centre 7, 8, 15, 16, 17, 21, 34, 41, 50, 58, 69, 80, 151–2, 157
London Lesbian and Gay Switchboard 1, 39, 187
London Lighthouse 162, 220

McCann, Patrick 31, 62, 65, 66, 67, 68–9, 70, 71, 89, 225
McClean, Sharley 212
McKellen, Sir Ian 9, 173
McKenna, Neil 67–8
Maclaine, Shirley 121
Madonna 62, 69
Major, John (MP) 113, 114, 117, 153, 167, 175, 176
March on Washington 147, 181
Mason, Angela 173, 182, 215
Mason, Michael 3, 16, 22, 26–7
Mayes, Steve 37, 53, 61, 77, 78, 84, 86, 88, 89, 91, 92, 93, 94, 103, 109, 113, 119, 122, 125, 129, 134, 135, 137, 140, 141, 148, 149, 151, 152, 153, 155, 156, 160, 168, 181, 183, 186, 191, 200

Maynard, Martin 108, 109, 110, 111, 121, 123, 124, 129, 133, 134, 136, 140, 176
Mellors, Bob 2
Melody Maker 143
Merck, Mandy 88
Mercury, Freddie 140, 143
Milligan, Don 25
Mirror 4, 113, 200
Morgan, David 153–4
Mugabe, Robert (President of Zimbabwe) 211
Muggeridge, Malcolm 2

National Gay and Lesbian Task Force (USA) 9, 182
National Viewers' and Listeners' Association 60–1, 138
Newsnight 201, 213

OLGA (Organization for Lesbian and Gay Action) 5, 6, 7, 21, 28
Oliver, Maureen 25
Organization for Lesbian and Gay Action, *see* OLGA
outing 63–71, 73, 184, 188, 189–92, 194–5, 197–202
Outweek 63, 143
Owolade, Alex 54

Paradise Club 34–5, 36, 54
'Paragraph 16' 50, 54
Parry, Will 171
Pink Paper 40, 129, 140, 150, 166, 227
Policing Initiative Group 37–41, 44, 83, 154–6, 166
Portillo, Michael (MP) 217, 218
Power, Lisa 4, 5, 6, 9, 10, 16, 24, 33, 35, 38, 42, 47, 51, 54, 56, 64, 122, 151, 172–3, 174, 176, 181, 224
Pride 22, 25, 41, 52, 154, 155, 180, 182, 217, 218, 225
Public Order Act 1986 31, 32, 164
PUSSY (Perverts Undermining State ScrutinY) 36, 87–8

QUANGO (Queer Accountants Never Go Out) 57, 129

QUARRELS (Queers Asserting the Right to Ride Every Line Safely) 90
queer 14–15, 55–8, 88, 90, 194, 219
Queer Accountants Never Go Out, *see* QUANGO
Queer Carnival 149–51
Queer Heritage 83, 184
Queer Nation (USA) 14, 15, 55, 57, 63, 73, 87
Queer Planet 91–2
Queer Reality 85–6
'Queer the Vote' 219–20
Queer Wedding 61–3, 110, 111
Queers Against Fundamentalism 186, 210
Queers Bash Back 96, 123–5, 215
QUID (Queers United In Dosh) 57, 82, 129

Radcliffe, Megan 36, 37, 55, 57, 78, 82, 88, 89, 90, 92, 93, 95, 96–7, 102, 122, 126, 128, 130, 225
Rank Outsiders 106, 107
Ranks, Shabba 145–6
Rawlston, Adam 22
RCP (Revolutionary Communist Party) 25, 26, 42, 43, 46
Reagan, Ronald (President of USA) 10
Revolutionary Communist Party, *see* RCP
Richard, Sir Cliff 2, 58–60
'Right-Off Caucus' 96
Robinson, Tom 109
Rodgerson, Gillian 16, 43
Rosetti, Gabriel 63–4
Royal Mail 140–1
Royal Television Society 147
Royal Tournament 123–4

Sainsbury's 205–6
Sanderson, Terry 105
Sandys, Sebastian 188, 189
Saunders, Jennifer 96–7, 128
Section 28, *see* Local Government Act 1988
Selleck, Tom 60, 67, 121, 140, 143, 154
Semple, Linda 43, 47

244 | Index

Sessional Orders 102, 103–4, 174
Sexual Offences Act 1956 108
SHAGPILES (Screaming Homos Against Gutless Prissy Icky Lawmakers Enforcing Celibacy) 57
Shea, Alan 80, 81
Signorile, Michelangelo 15, 63, 66, 143
Silence of the Lambs 144
Sinitta 155
SISSY (Sex Information for Schools, Students and Youth) 98–100
Sisters of Perpetual Indulgence 32, 47, 51, 55, 59, 79, 118, 122, 137, 138, 140, 168, 172, 173
SLAGS (Socialist Lesbians And Gays) 84–5
Sky TV 44
Slater, Douglas 51
Smith, Cherry 97
Smith, Chris (MP) 197, 215
Smith, John (MP) 177, 178, 179
Socialist Lesbians and Gays, *see* SLAGS
Somerville, Jimmy 52, 104, 109
Spanner trial 50–1, 138, 146
Spence, Christopher 172–3
Square Peg 32
Stannard, Steve 17, 22, 23, 26, 33, 36, 40, 43, 44, 45, 46, 84, 85, 226–7
Stone, Sharon 144

Stonewall Group 9–10, 16, 38, 39, 42, 51, 67, 85, 99, 106, 154, 168, 171, 172, 173, 181, 182, 194, 197, 209, 210, 211, 220, 224
Stuart, Dr Elizabeth 139
Summerskill, Ben 150
Sun 60, 67, 121, 140, 143, 154
Sunday Times 65, 66
Sutcliffe, Lynne 33, 37, 62, 63, 64, 76, 89, 90, 91, 95, 98, 111, 113–14, 121, 122, 129, 135, 138, 146, 151, 160, 166, 169, 174, 179, 180, 181, 224–5

Tatchell, Peter 3, 5, 8, 15, 16, 17, 18, 30, 26, 32, 33, 38, 39, 41, 45–6, 54, 56, 59, 64, 65, 66, 67, 68, 70, 81, 92, 93, 94, 97, 101, 118, 129, 134, 146, 147, 154, 155, 156, 167, 168, 169, 174, 175, 176, 186, 187, 188, 189, 190, 191, 194, 195, 198, 200, 201, 206, 211, 212, 213, 214, 215, 216, 217, 225–6, 228, 236–40
Taylor, John (Bishop of St Albans) 204–5
Tebbit, Norman (MP) 50
Teresa, Mother 27
Terrence Higgins Trust 28, 162, 168
Thatcher, Baroness Margaret 5, 10, 105
Time Out 52, 117
Top of the Pops 145–6
True Freedom Trust 202, 203, 205

Tuesday Group 103, 119, 127
Turnbull, Michael (Archbishop of Durham) 188–9
Tutu, Desmond (Archbishop of Cape Town) 25

Vatican Embassy 133–5
Vauxhall Tavern 90
Vibewatchers 57, 130, 139
Village Soho 124, 149

Wallace, Neil 46, 54
Walter, Aubrey 2
Watney, Simon 8, 10, 13, 15, 16, 19, 20, 23, 25, 26, 34–5, 43, 44, 45, 216, 226
Watson, Oscar 21
Watts, Steven 140–1
whistles 23–5, 32
White, Chris 58
White, Jenny 60
Whitehouse, Mary 2, 27, 60–1
Whores of Babylon 73–80, 87
WIG (Work It Girl) 88–90, 168
Wilde, Oscar 52
Wilshire, David (MP) 5, 28
Winter Pride, *see* Pride
Winterton, Ann (MP) 19
Woods, Chris 3, 15, 16, 20, 31, 34, 36, 39, 41, 43, 44, 45, 51, 53, 56, 57, 58, 63, 64, 70, 91, 102, 124, 130, 161, 227

YOUTH (Young radical queers Ostracizing Ubiquitous Tyrannical Heterosexism) 99–100, 127